Free with

BD Chaurasia's

Human Anatomy | Volum

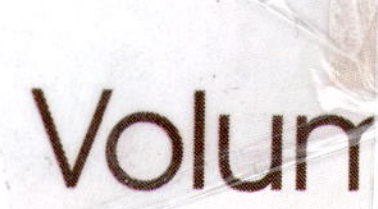

Tenth Edition

Workbook of Human Anatomy

Learn | Assess | Practice Activity

As per the latest NMC Guidelines | Competency Based Medical Education (CBME) Curriculum under Graduate Medical Education Regulation

Upper Limb

Thorax

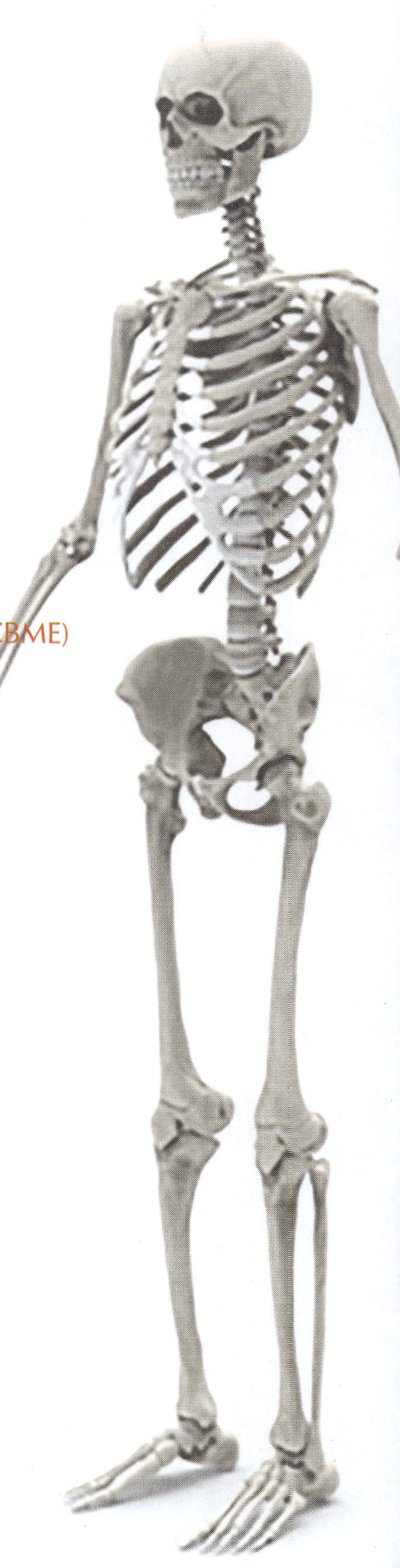

Free with

BD Chaurasia's

Human Anatomy | Volume 1

Tenth Edition

Workbook of Human Anatomy

Learn | Assess | Practice Activity

As per the latest NMC Guidelines | Competency Based Medical Education (CBME) Curriculum under Graduate Medical Education Regulation

Upper Limb

Thorax

Executive Editor, BD Chaurasia's *Human Anatomy*, Tenth Edition

Yogesh Ashok Sontakke MBBS MD

Additional Professor

Department of Anatomy

Jawaharlal Institute of Postgraduate Medical Education and Research (JIPMER)

(An Institute of National Importance under the Ministry of Health and Family Welfare, Government of India)

Puducherry, India

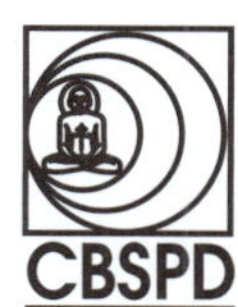

CBS Publishers & Distributors Pvt Ltd

New Delhi • Bengaluru • Chennai • Kochi • Kolkata • Lucknow • Mumbai

Hyderabad • Jharkhand • Nagpur • Patna • Pune • Uttarakhand

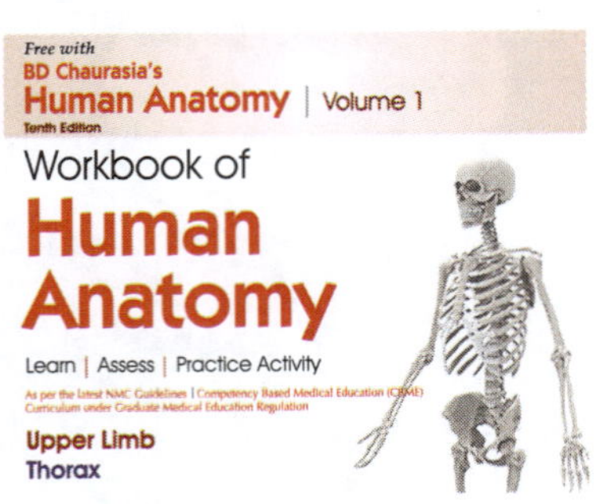

To accompany BD Chaurasia's Human Anatomy Vol 1

ISBN: 978-93-5466-979-8

Published by Satish Kumar Jain and produced by Varun Jain for

CBS Publishers & Distributors Pvt Ltd
4819/XI Prahlad Street, 24 Ansari Road, Daryaganj, New Delhi 110 002, India
Ph: 011-23289259, 23266838 Website: www.cbspd.com
e-mail: delhi@cbspd.com

Corporate Office: 204 FIE, Industrial Area, Patparganj, Delhi 110 092, India
Ph: 011-4934 4934 Fax: 011-4934 4935 e-mail: publishing@cbspd.com; publicity@cbspd.com

Branches

- **Bengaluru:** Seema House 2975, 17th Cross, K.R. Road, Banasankari 2nd Stage, Bengaluru 560 070, Karnataka, India
Ph: +91-80-26771678/79 Fax: +91-80-26771680 e-mail: bangalore@cbspd.com
- **Chennai:** 18/8B, Subbarayan Street, Shenoy Nagar, Chennai 600 030, Tamil Nadu, India
Ph: +91-44-42032115, 26681266 e-mail: chennai@cbspd.com
- **Kochi:** 42/1325, 1326, Power House Road, Opposite KSEB, Power House, Ernakulum 682018, Kochi, Kerala, India
Ph: +91-484-4059061–65, 67 Fax: +91-484-4059065 e-mail: kochi@cbspd.com
- **Kolkata:** 147, Hind Ceramics Compound, 1st Floor, Nilgunj Road, Belghoria, Kolkata 700056, West Bengal, India
Ph: +91-33-25633055/56 e-mail: kolkata@cbspd.com
- **Lucknow:** Basement, Khushnuma Complex, 7 Meerabai Marg (behind Jawahar Bhawan), Lucknow 226001, UP, India
Ph: +91-522-4000032 e-mail: tiwari.lucknow@cbspd.com
- **Mumbai:** PWD Shed, Gala No. 25/26, Ramchandra Bhatt Marg, Next JJ Hospital Gate No. 2, Opp. Union Bank of India, Noorbaug, Mumbai 400009, Maharashtra, India
Ph: +91-22-66661880/89 e-mail: mumbai@cbspd.com

Representatives

- **Hyderabad** 0-9885175004
- **Jharkhand** 0-9811541605
- **Nagpur** 0-8692091830
- **Patna** 0-9334159340
- **Pune** 0-9664372571
- **Uttarakhand** 0-9716462459

Printed at: Thomson Press (India) Ltd., Faridabad, Haryana, India

Preface

The *Workbook of Human Anatomy* is prepared after discussions with the students to fulfil the requirements of students for examination preparations. This workbook will help the students to achieve the required levels of the given competencies: Knows (K), knows how (KH) and shows how (SH), with the help of included domains of learning, knowledge (K) and skills (S). To fulfil the need for curriculum, requirements of the students and the field of medicine, it is essential for every learner to convert subject knowledge into presentable format in the examinations.

Students face the problem in revision and focusing on the practice of figures and revising the subject. Each book on the anatomy contains thousands of images. It is very difficult to select the figures to be practised. To solve these students' concerns, this *Workbook* has been prepared to help the students by making them aware about practising selected figures for preparation of theory examinations. The students should keep in mind that while answering the questions in the examination about anatomy, if they support the answer by a selected figure, the explanation will be easy and presentable.

To address these issues of the students, this workbook is facilitated with the following features:

1. Clinicoanatomical problems will help to sensitize the students to Early Clinical Exposure.
2. MCQs will help in analysing the understanding of the subject.
3. Question Bank will help to prepare for upcoming academic examinations.
4. Spotters will help to prepare for practical examinations.
5. Answer Keys will help to cross-check and self-assessments.

Always read a complete textbook for getting better knowledge and generating perfect concepts of the subject. ***Cadavers and dissections are the best teachers of human anatomy***. Due to increasing number of students in the medical colleges and less availability of cadavers, under the expertise of teachers, the students can utilize their spare time in the dissection hall to complete this workbook. It will help in consolidation of the knowledge and better understanding of the structures. Due to space constrain, all practice figures are not included in this Workbook. Students are advised to practice additional images in their practice notebooks.

For any suggestions, please write at dryogeshas@gmail.com

Yogesh Ashok Sontakke
dryogeshas@gmail.com

Instructions to Students

1. Read the theory part from the main textbook before starting to solve the workbook.
2. *Clinicoanatomical problems*: Read these problems carefully. Write precise answers. Use separate sheet of copy for writing in details.
3. *Practice figures*: As we are aware that many students are good in drawings and to avoid difficulty of initial stages of drawings, the workbook is provided with dotted outlines of practice figures. Trace these lines with suitable colour pencils and shade the figures. Refer the main Textbook before colouring the figures. Label the figures with good handwriting.
4. *MCQs*: Tick the single best correct option in the workbook. Some diagram based MCQs are introduced to align with CBME pattern.
5. *Question Bank*: It will give orientation towards upcoming academic examinations. Use separate copy to solve the following questions. Maintain this copy properly so that it can be referred during subject revision.
6. *Spotters*: These will give orientation towards practical examinations. Solve them on a separate sheet.
7. *Answer Keys*: Match your answers with the provided key. Self-evaluation is the best method for progress.
8. *eSmartQuiz – Online MCQ test*: Scan the QR code for online MCQ test. Fill the required details and solve the test.

   Always keep in mind "*Practice is essential and integral part of academics. Hard work is the path for success*".

Yogesh Ashok Sontakke

Contents

eSmartQuiz – Online MCQ Test

After attending the class, students should go through the "*eSmartQuiz* – Online MCQ test" for the following reasons:

- *Reinforcement of Learning*: The "*eSmartQuiz* – Online MCQ test" provides an opportunity to reinforce learning after attending a class or reading a book. It helps to assess understanding and retention of concepts, to solidify knowledge and identify areas that need further revision or clarification.
- *Assessment of Comprehension*: The "*eSmartQuiz* – Online MCQ test" is an effective tool to assess comprehension of the subject matter and to demonstrate the ability to apply the concepts learned in the class.
- *Enhancement of Attention and Critical Thinking*: The "*eSmartQuiz* – Online MCQ test" will help to make students attentive for the class and to enhance critical thinking skills by selecting the most appropriate answer among the given options.

Each *eSmartQuiz* test consists of 10 MCQs, mostly image-based, and the students can see their scores at the end of each test. These questions will be modified after a certain interval. Use the given links or scan the QR code (given in each chapter) for the test. One student can solve each test only one time.

Chapter	*Link for* ***eSmartQuiz***
Upper Limb	
1. Introduction	https://forms.gle/cbNoHpx1AZ1Cci3WA
2. Bones	https://forms.gle/BNwB1uVpZ3QkKH3LA
3. Pectoral Region	https://forms.gle/2uvWyFGqwH58Aqgc9
4. Axilla	https://forms.gle/tn4WgHoLYpHZMkGp9
5. Back	https://forms.gle/eV9AjxwFU8bvDVRp6
6. Scapular Region	https://forms.gle/LHZ9MCB8r8pwJjfM6
7. Cutaneous Nerves, Superficial Veins and Lymphatic Drainage	https://forms.gle/nvVW9dhwfkLpNmHA8
8. Arm	https://forms.gle/q9G441mXn6e7D5YA9
9. Forearm and Hand	https://forms.gle/TD47GgMsajUsaKbP7
10. Joints of Upper Limb	https://forms.gle/Uz58AQZEBoV8jC2V6
11. Surface Marking and Radiological Anatomy of Upper Limb	https://forms.gle/pFqy9AdXNZU9WnJa6
Thorax	
12. Introduction	https://forms.gle/JmnZB66BgAFrQGgz5
13. Bones and Joints of Thorax	https://forms.gle/dsP6Ps5dw7sk3xYw5
14. Walls of Thorax	https://forms.gle/YZUu7n85AzWVqKEt6
15. Thoracic Cavity and Pleurae	https://forms.gle/uqdyCGyqE765sxFK6
16. Lungs	https://forms.gle/n7zigPn8smjNhTbD7
17. Mediastinum	https://forms.gle/RbeqSJKtANvFu6ay9
18. Pericardium and Heart	https://forms.gle/qys5zAdbsMTrNNSs8
19. Superior Vena Cava, Aorta and Pulmonary Trunk	https://forms.gle/ZDEkSQRMBM2H7mPf8
20. Trachea, Oesophagus and Thoracic Duct	https://forms.gle/CYwJap1ASNUaQpkQ9
21. Surface Marking and Radiological Anatomy of Thorax	https://forms.gle/PmCLumZeqdWXiPWx5

Upper Limb

Chapter

1

eSmartQuiz

Introduction

PRACTICE FIGURES

(Label the practice figures)

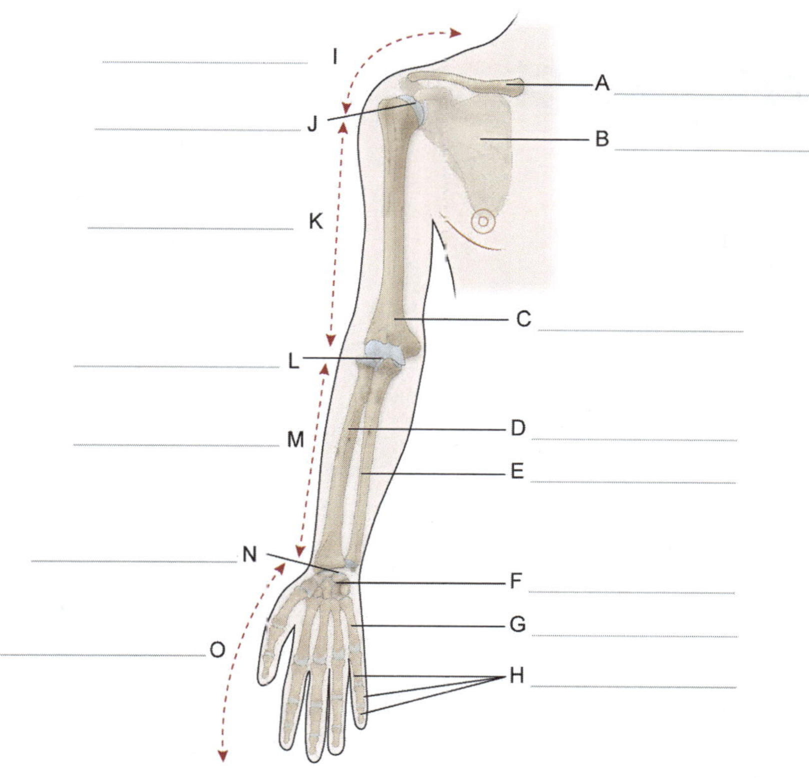

Practice Figure 1.1: Parts and bones of upper limb

A. Name of the instrument: ____________________

24

4

B ____________________

C ____________________

D ____________________

E. Uses: ____________________

Practice Figure 1.2: Name the instrument and its parts and uses

A. Name of the instrument: ____________

B. Uses: ____________

C. Name of the instrument: ____________

D. Uses: ____________

E. Name of the instrument: ____________

F. Uses: ____________

Practice Figure 1.3: Name the instrument and mention its uses

MULTIPLE CHOICE QUESTIONS

(Tick the single best correct option)

1. What is antebrachium?
   a. Shoulder b. Arm
   c. Forearm d. Hand
2. ____________ is the bone of arm.
   a. Clavicle b. Scapula
   c. Humerus d. Radius
3. Wrist is supported by ____________ carpal bones.
   a. 6 b. 7
   c. 8 d. 9
4. Which of the following joints is formed by the radius bone?
   a. Elbow b. Superior radioulnar
   c. Inferior radioulnar d. All of the above
5. Thumb has ____________ interphalangeal joint/s.
   a. 0 b. 1
   c. 2 d. 3
6. Which of the following is true regarding the force of weight transmission in the upper limb?
   a. Transferred from radius to ulna
   b. Transferred from scapula to vertebral column
   c. Transferred from scapula to humerus
   d. Transferred from radius to humerus
7. Which of the following is true regarding the upper limb in comparison with the lower limb?
   a. Presence of a carrying angle
   b. Supination and pronation movements
   c. Opposition actions of thumb
   d. All of the above
8. Identify the following instrument.

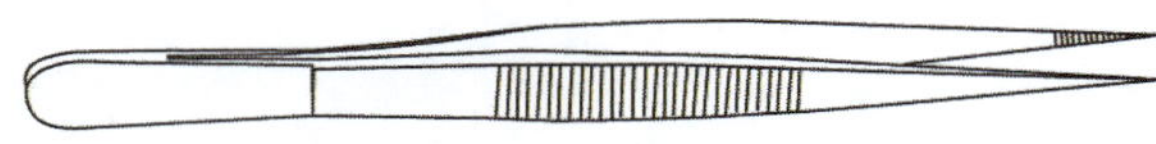

   a. Plane forceps b. Artery forceps
   c. Pointed forceps d. Toothed forceps
9. Identify the following instrument.

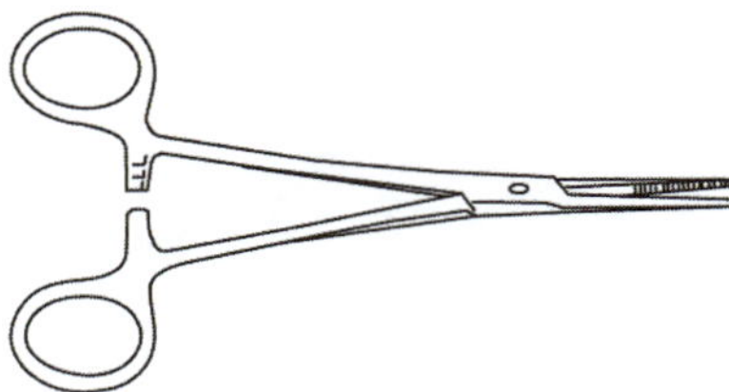

   a. Plane forceps b. Artery forceps
   c. Pointed forceps d. Toothed forceps
10. Identify the following instrument.

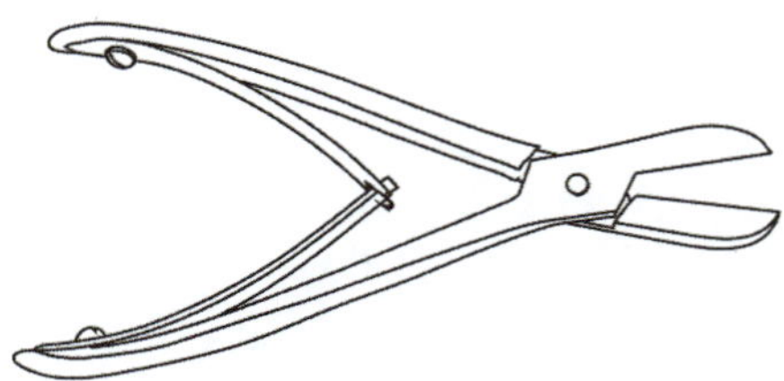

   a. Bone nibbler b. Surgical chisel
   c. Surgical blade d. Haemostatic forceps
11. Which of the following cadaveric structures has a cord-like feel?
   a. Artery b. Vein
   c. Nerve d. Lymph node

QUESTION BANK

(Use separate copy to solve the following questions)

Q 1. Mention the path for lines of force transmission in the upper limb.

Q 2. Name the homologous parts of the upper and lower limbs.

Q 3. Enumerate:
   a. Subdivisions of shoulder region
   b. Joints of the forearm
   c. Joints of the hand

eSmartQuiz

Bones

CLINICOANATOMICAL PROBLEMS

Clinical Case 1

A 50-year-old man fell off his bicycle. He heard a cracking noise and felt severe pain in his right shoulder region. He noted that the lateral part of the shoulder drooped and medial end of clavicle was elevated.

Q 1. Which is the common site of fracture of clavicle and why?
Q 2. Why did his shoulder droop down?

Explanation

1. ______________________________

2. ______________________________

Clinical Case 2

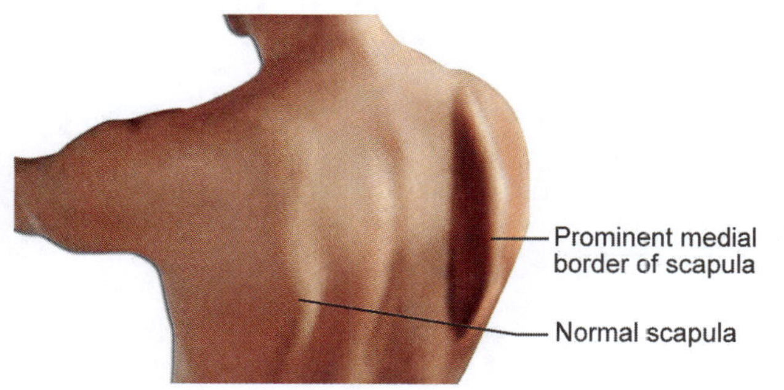

Q 1. Identify the clinical condition shown in the above figure.
Q 2. Name the part of the bone which became prominent and why?

Explanation

1. ______________________________

2. ______________________________

Clinical Case 3

A 30-year-old male had a history of falling on his left shoulder while playing and presented with swelling at the junction of neck and shoulder. Patient is holding the affected arm in adducted position close to body. On examination, it is observed that shoulder is in typically pulled downwards position.

Q 1. Identify the clinical condition.
Q 2. What has happened with the bones in this condition?

Explanation

1. ______________________________

2. ______________________________

Clinical Case 4

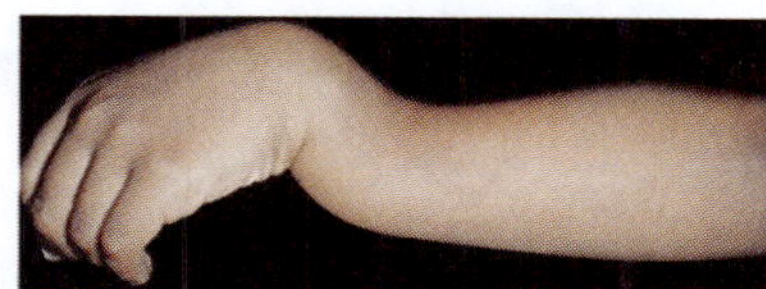

A 35-year-old woman presents to the emergency department after a fall on an outstretched hand. She complains of severe pain in her left wrist. On physical examination, swelling, tenderness and deformity at the left wrist were found. The patient showed the following appearance of the lower part of the forearm and hand.

Q 1. What deformity is shown in the above image?
Q 2. What is the anatomical basis for this finding?
Q 3. Which investigation do you suggest for the confirmation of your diagnosis?

Explanation

1. ______________________________

2. ______________________________

3. ______________________________

PRACTICE FIGURES

(Colour and label the practice figures. Use suitable colour codes)

(a) Superior view
F
A
E
B
(b) Inferior view
E
C
D
J
H
I
G

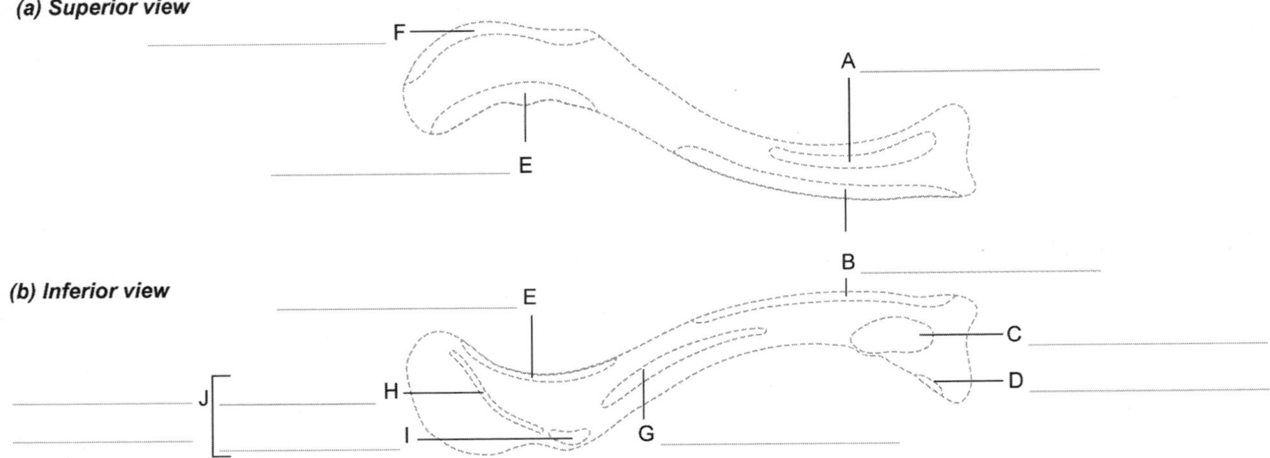

Practice Figure 2.1: Attachments of clavicle

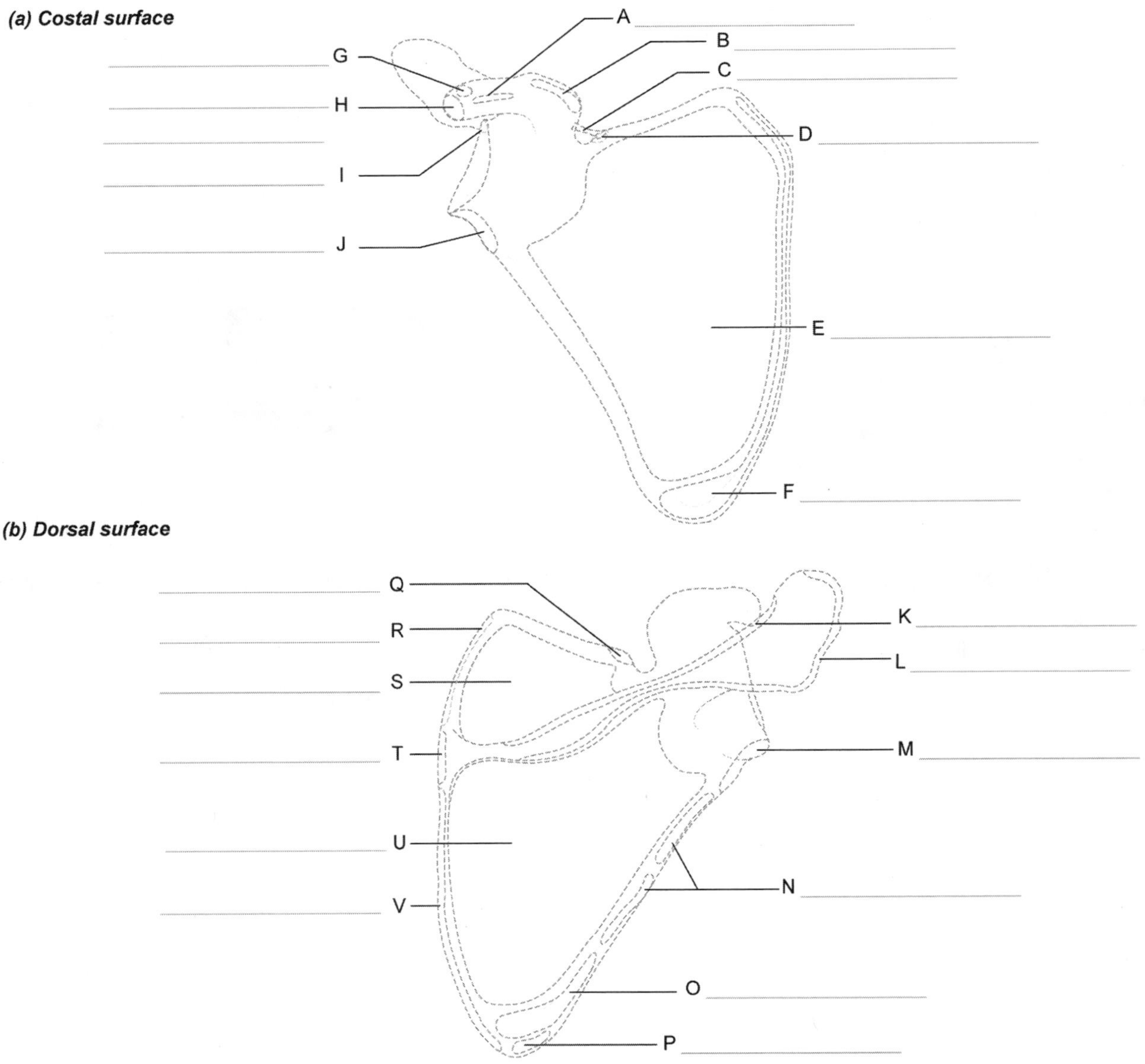

(a) Costal surface
A
B
C
G
H
D
I
J
E
F
(b) Dorsal surface
Q
R
S
T
U
V
K
L
M
N
O
P

Practice Figure 2.2: Attachments of scapula

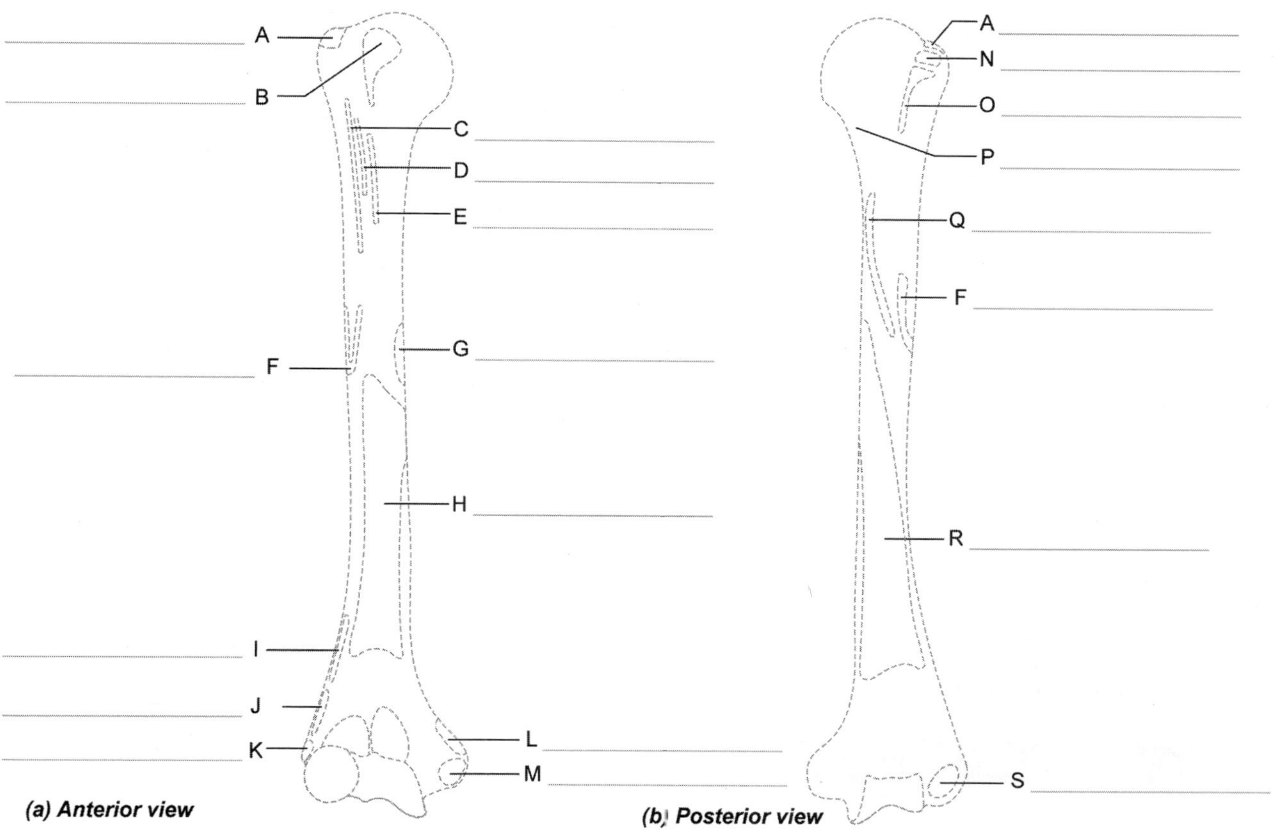

Practice Figure 2.3: Attachments of humerus: (a) Anterior view and (b) posterior view

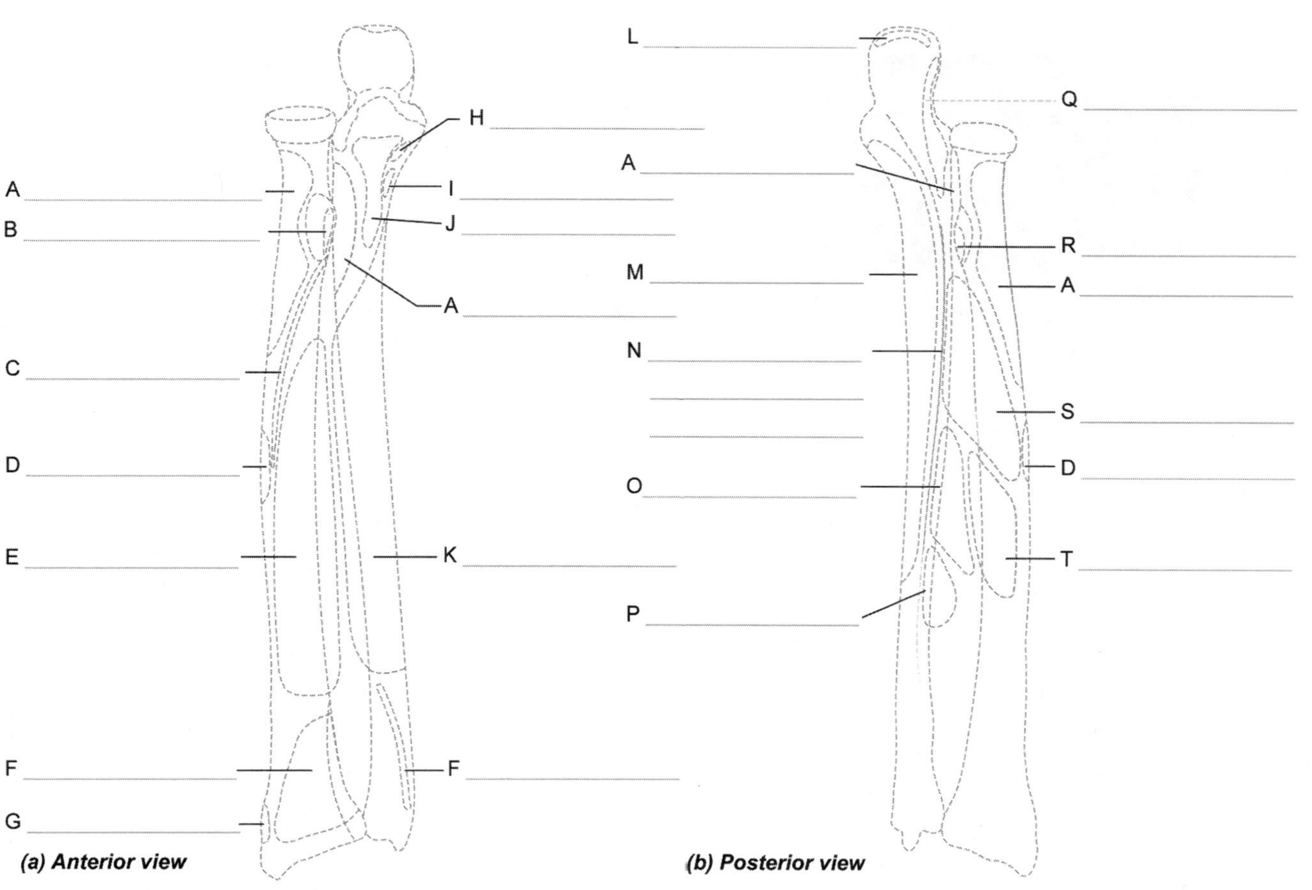

Practice Figure 2.4: Attachments of radius and ulna: (a) Anterior aspect and (b) Posterior aspect

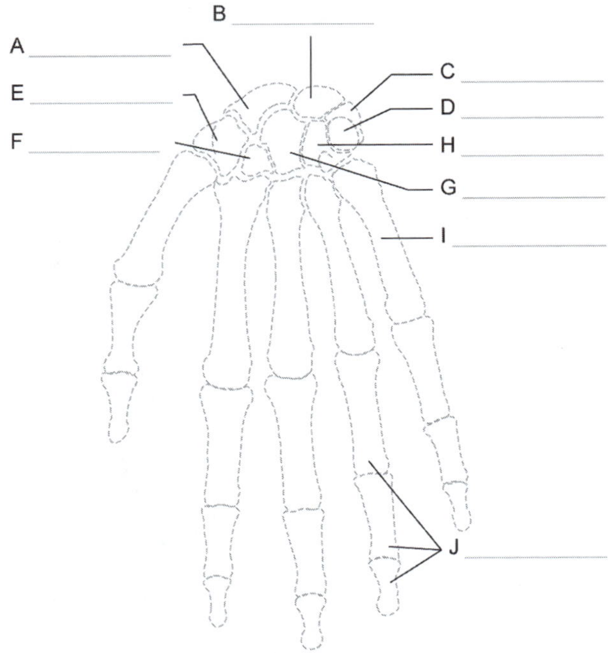

Practice Figure 2.5: Bones of hand

MULTIPLE CHOICE QUESTIONS

(Tick the single best correct option)

1. Fall on an outstretched hand causes all these conditions, EXCEPT:
   a. Dislocation of shoulder
   b. Colles' fracture
   c. Fracture of scaphoid
   d. Smith's fracture
2. Identify the fractured bone in the following X-ray.

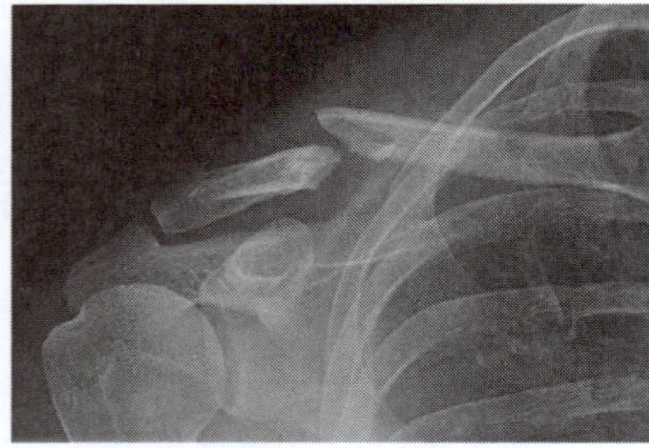

   a. Clavicle b. Coracoid process
   c. Humerus d. Ribs
3. All of the following muscles are attached to the coracoid process of scapula, EXCEPT:
   a. Biceps brachii b. Coracobrachialis
   c. Triceps brachii d. Pectoralis minor
4. Transverse head of adductor pollicis muscle originates from ____________ metacarpal.
   a. Second metacarpal b. Third metacarpal
   c. Fourth metacarpal d. Fifth metacarpal
5. Buddy split is useful for the treatment of fractures of the ____________.
   a. Scapula b. Humerus
   c. Metacarpal d. Phalanx
6. Which of the following carpal undergoes avascular necrosis in its fracture?
   a. Scaphoid b. Lunate
   c. Triquetrum d. Pisiform
7. Colles' fracture is a fracture of ____________ bone.
   a. Clavicle b. Humerus
   c. Radius d. Ulna
8. Which of the following bones is the first one to start ossification?
   a. Clavicle b. Humerus
   c. Radius d. Ulna
9. All of the following nerves are related to the humerus, EXCEPT:
   a. Axillary b. Radial
   c. Ulnar d. Musculocutaneous
10. Which of the following muscles is attached to the medial lip of the bicipital groove?
   a. Pectoralis major b. Latissimus dorsi
   c. Teres major d. Teres minor
11. Identify the carpal (i) and (ii).

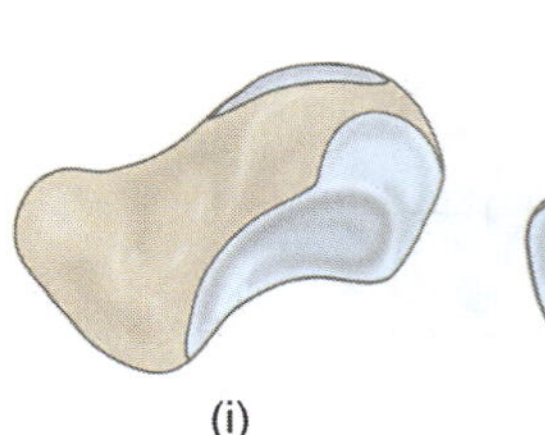

(i)

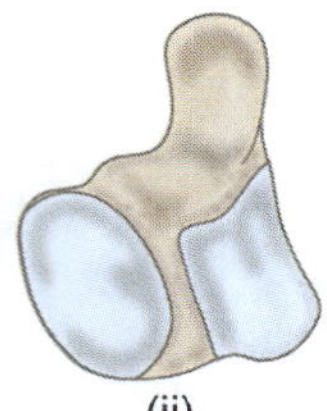

(ii)

   a. Scaphoid, triquetrum
   b. Scaphoid, hamate
   c. Lunate, capitate
   d. Trapezoid, hamate
12. Identify the structure X.

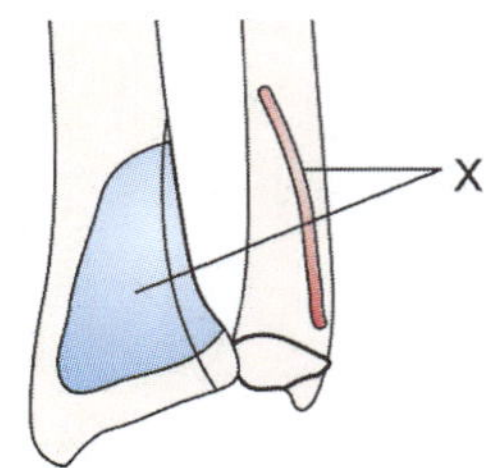

   a. Pronator teres b. Brachioradialis
   c. Flexor pollicis longus d. Pronator quadratus

DISSECTION AND PRACTICAL QUESTIONS

Q. Determine the side and hold the following bones in anatomical positions:

A. Clavicle B. Scapula
C. Humerus D. Radius
E. Ulna

QUESTION BANK

(Use separate copy to solve the following questions)

Q 1. List the peculiarities of clavicle.
Q 2. Mention the features of coracoid process of scapula.
Q 3. Name the muscles attached to the medial border of scapula.
Q 4. List the nerve closely related to humerus.
Q 5. Write a short note on supracondylar fracture of humerus.
Q 6. List the peculiarities of pisiform bone.
Q 7. Explain the anatomical basis of avascular necrosis of scaphoid fracture.

eSmartQuiz

Pectoral Region

CLINICOANATOMICAL PROBLEMS

Clinical Case 1

A 50-year-old female patient came to the OPD. She had a complaint of blood discharge from the right nipple since 1 month. On clinical examination, a firm, non-tender, 2 × 2 cm mass was found in the upper lateral quadrant of her right breast. The nipple was retracted, and blood discharge came out in gentle squeezing. The clinician suspected her as a case of breast cancer.

Q 1. Which lymph nodes should be palpated by the clinician and why?
Q 2. What causes the retraction of the nipple?
Q 3. Which radiological investigation will help with the diagnosis?

Explanation

1.
2.
3.

Clinical Case 2

A 45-year-old female patient visited a tertiary care hospital for the complaint of a painless lump in her left breast. On clinical examination, the physician found the following findings. Give the anatomical reasons for each of these findings.

1. Hard lump of 3 × 3 cm in upper outer quadrant
2. Peau d'orange appearance of the skin
3. Loss of mobility of breast
4. Enlargement of axillary lymph nodes
5. X-ray of vertebral column: Irregular shadow in the vertebral bodies of T3 and T6 vertebrae.

Explanation

1.
2.
3.
4.
5.

Clinical Case 3

For clinical testing of a pectoralis major muscle, the clinician had asked the patient to perform the following activity.

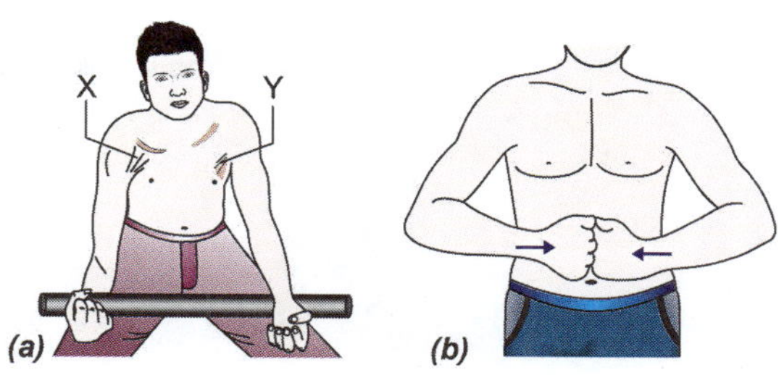

Based on it, name the part of the pectoralis major muscle tested clinically.

1. X part in figure a
2. Y part in figure a
3. Part of the muscle in figure b.

Explanation

1.
2.
3.

Clinical Case 4

A 25-year-old watchman protected the house from thieves. He got injured on the right lateral wall of the chest. On clinical examination, when the clinician asked to push a wall, the medial border of the right scapula became prominent (shown in the adjacent figure).

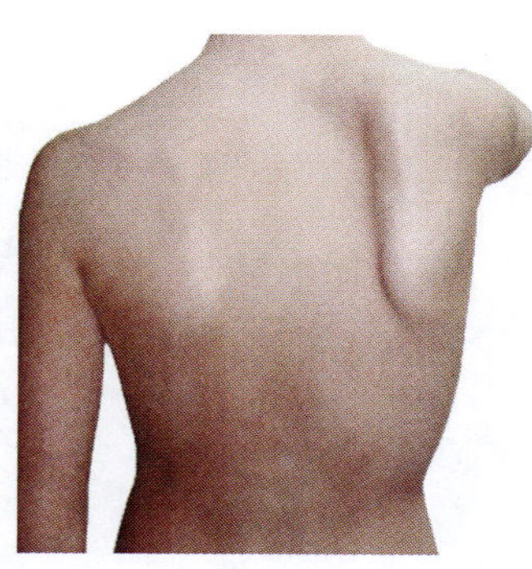

Q 1. Identify the clinical condition shown in the figure.
Q 2. Why did the medial border of the scapula become prominent in this case?

Explanation

1.

2.

PRACTICE FIGURES

(Colour and label the practice figures. Use suitable colour codes)

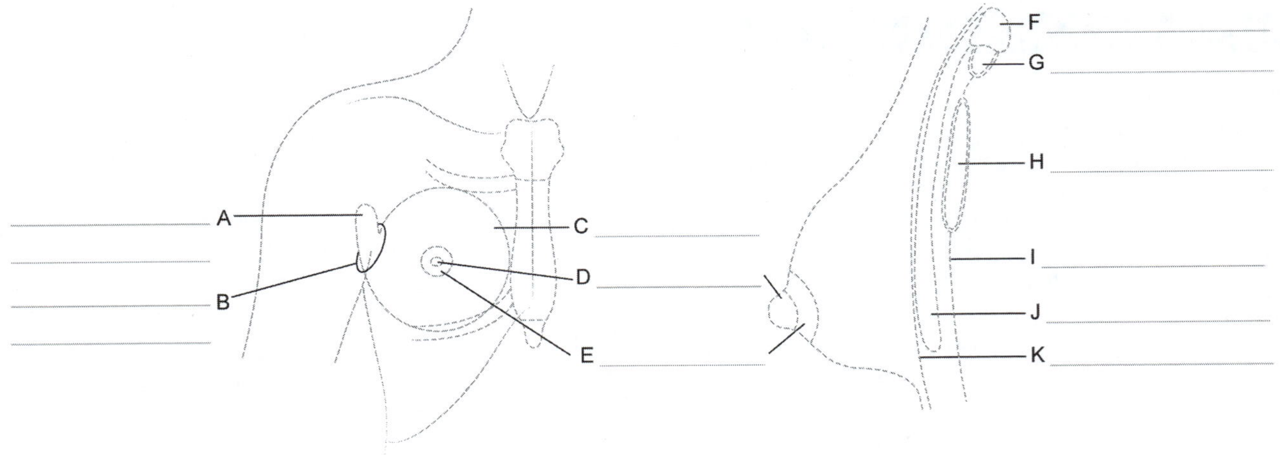

Practice Figure 3.1: Parts and deep relations of breast

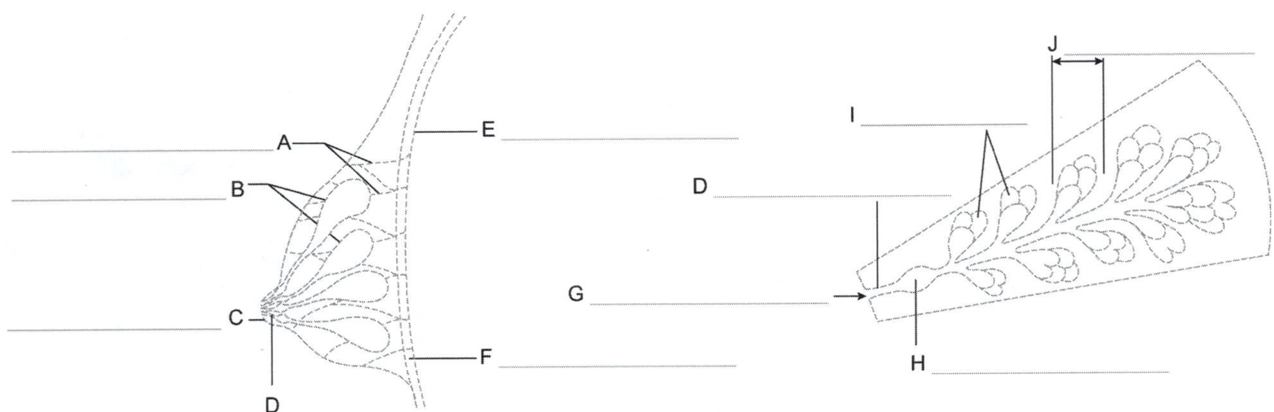

Practice Figure 3.2: Structure of breast and its lobule

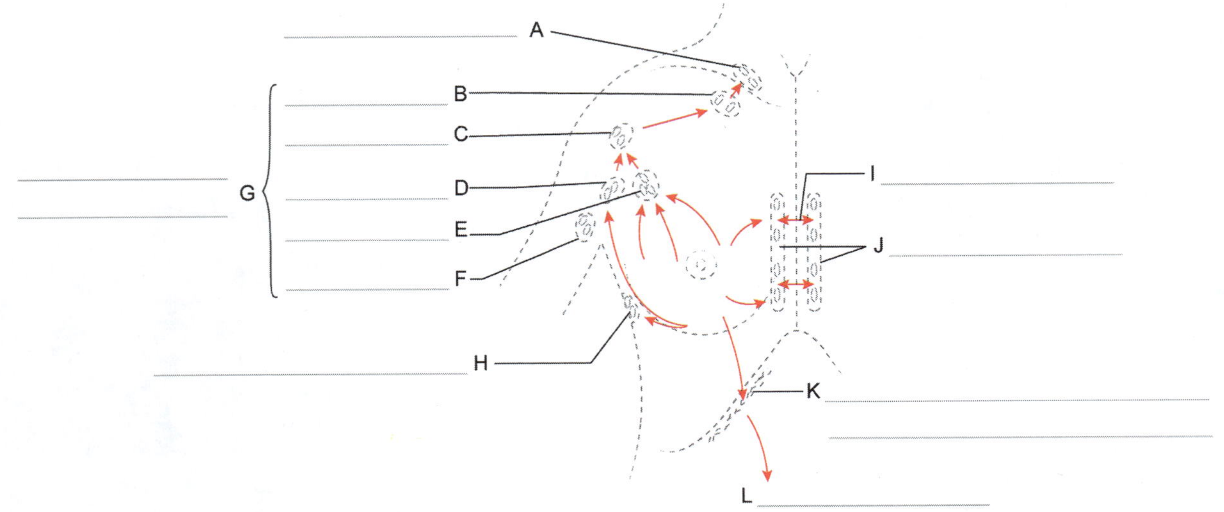

Practice Figure 3.3: Lymphatic drainage of breast

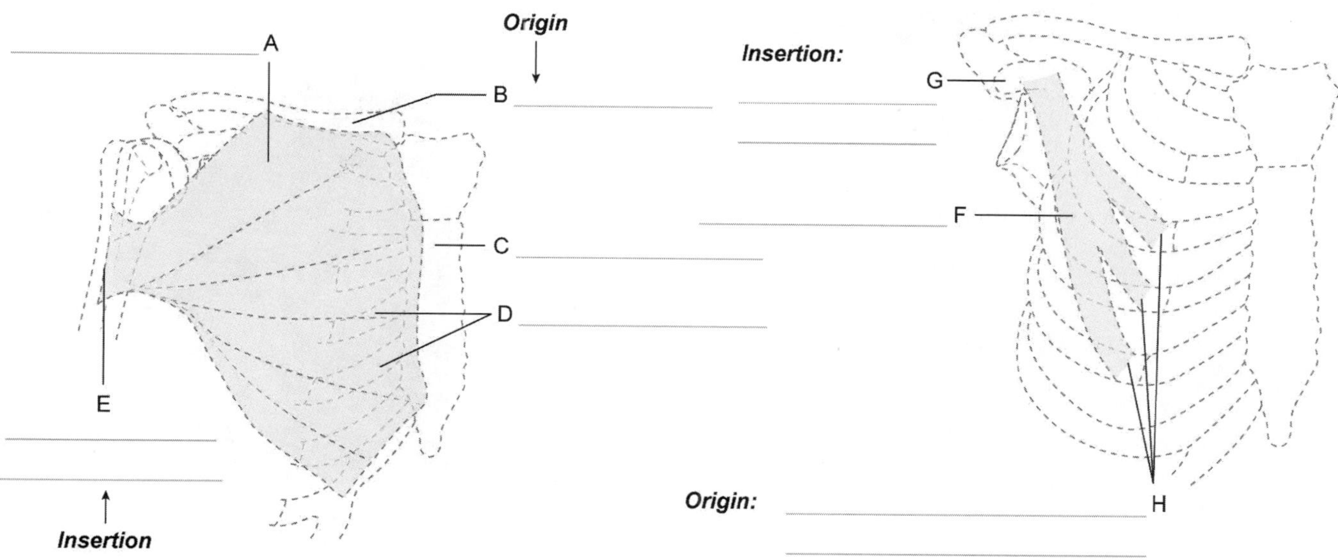

Practice Figure 3.4: Pectoralis major and minor muscles

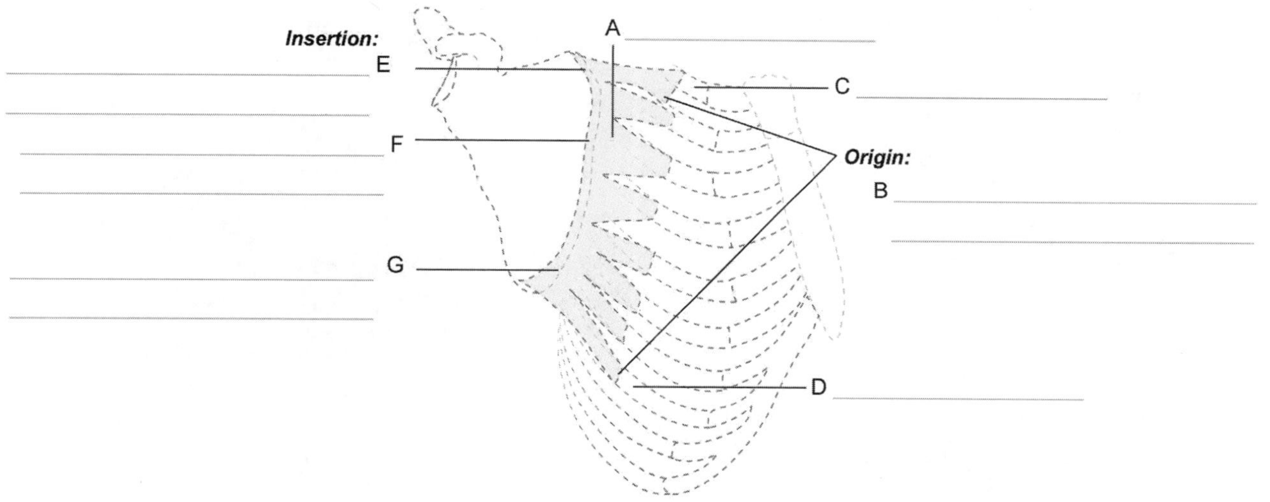

Practice Figure 3.5: Serratus anterior muscle

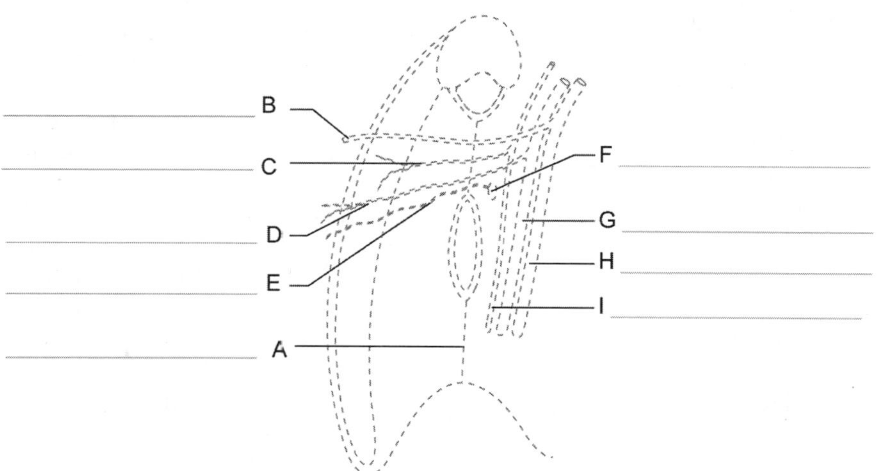

Practice Figure 3.6: Structures piercing clavipectoral fascia

MULTIPLE CHOICE QUESTIONS

(Tick the single best correct option)

1. Mammary gland is a modified ____________.
   a. Apocrine sweat gland b. Eccrine sweat gland
   c. Sebaceous gland d. Serous gland
2. All of the following structures pierce the clavipectoral fascia, EXCEPT:
   a. Cephalic vein b. Thoracoacromial artery
   c. Axillary vein d. Lateral pectoral nerve
3. ____________ muscle is present within the clavipectoral fascia.
   a. Pectoralis major b. Pectoralis minor
   c. Serratus anterior d. Sternocleidomastoid
4. All of the following muscles are related to the deep surface of the mammary gland, EXCEPT:
   a. Pectoralis major
   b. Pectoralis minor
   c. Serratus anterior
   d. Sternocleidomastoid
5. Most of the lymph from breast is drained into the ____________ axillary lymph nodes.
   a. Anterior b. Posterior
   c. Lateral d. Apical
6. Line of Schultz appears during the ____________ week of intrauterine life.
   a. 3rd b. 6th
   c. 8th d. 10th
7. Rotter's lymph nodes are ____________ nodes.
   a. Interpectoral b. Apical axillary
   c. Internal thoracic d. Supraclavicular
8. The most common site of the breast cancer is ____________ quadrant.
   a. Upper inner b. Upper outer
   c. Lower inner d. Lower outer
9. The lymphatic plexus of Sappey is located in which part of the breast?
   a. Areola b. Lobes
   c. Stoma d. Acini
10. Identify the structure X and Y shown in the following figures.

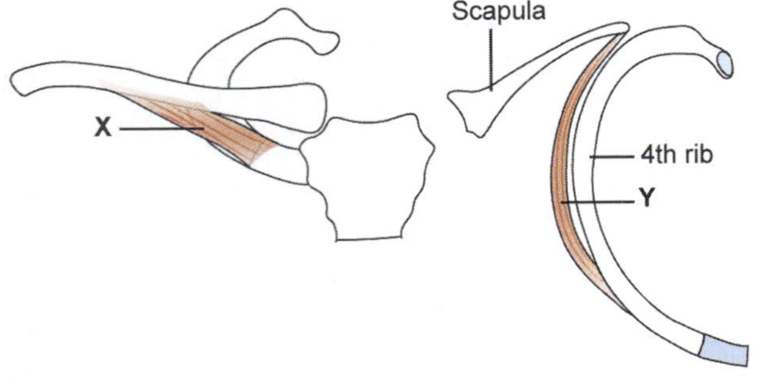

   a. Pectoralis minor, serratus anterior
   b. Serratus anterior, subclavius
   c. Subclavius, serratus anterior
   d. Subclavius, pectoralis minor
11. What is the use of the radiograph shown in the following figure?

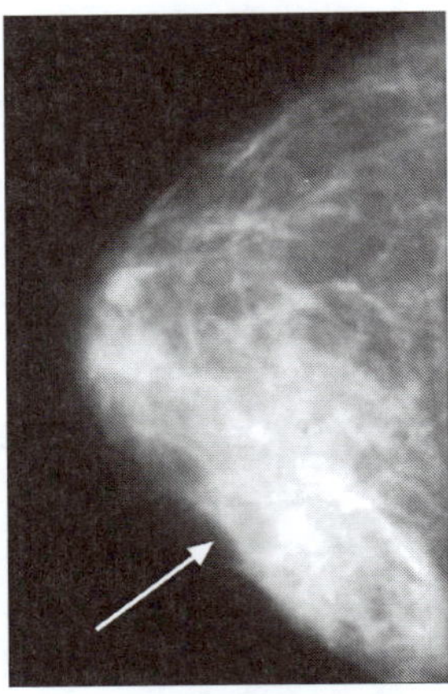

   a. Detection of fracture of clavicle
   b. Detection lung cancer
   c. Detection of breast cancer
   d. Detection of tumour of pectoralis major
12. Name the condition shown in the following figure.

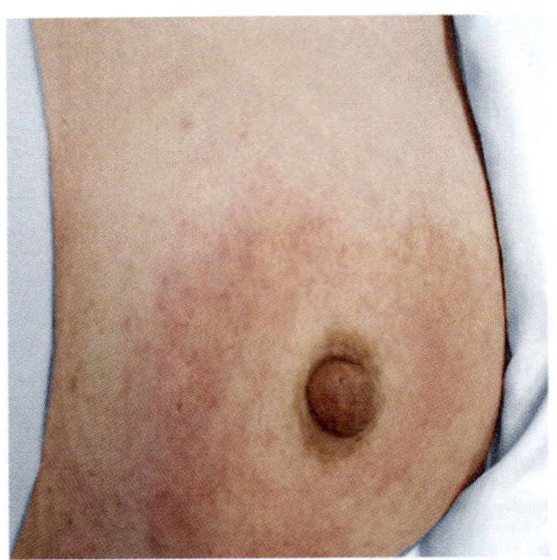

   a. Retraction of nipple
   b. Retraction of skin
   c. Lump in the breast
   d. Peau d'orange appearance

QUESTION BANK

(Use separate copy to solve the following questions)

Q 1. Describe the mammary gland under the following heads: Location, extent, morphology, structure, external features, relations, blood supply and nerve supply.

Q 2. Write a short note:
   a. Applied aspects of mammary gland.
   b. Lymphatic drainage of breast.
   c. Clavipectoral fascia.

Q 3. List the structures piercing clavipectoral fascia.

Q 4. Explain the anatomical basis of:
   a. Metastasis from carcinoma of inferomedial quadrant of breast may take place in pelvic cavity or Krukenberg's tumour.
   b. Retraction and puckering of skin of breast.
   c. The peau d'orange, and retraction of nipple.
   d. Winging of scapula.

eSmartQuiz

Axilla

CLINICOANATOMICAL PROBLEMS

Clinical Case 1

Kranti, a one and half-year-old baby, is brought to the pediatrician by her parents. They noticed that Kranti seemed to have difficulty moving her right arm. Upon examination, the pediatrician observed that Kranti had inability to abduct the right shoulder (Finding a). Kranti struggled to bend her right elbow (Finding b). Kranti's right forearm remains in a fixed position with the palm facing downward (Finding c). Kranti's mother reported difficult delivery. The pediatrician diagnosed Kranti with Erb's palsy.

1. What structure had damage in Kranti?
2. What are the anatomical reasons for Findings a, b and c.

Explanation

1. ______________________________

____

____

2. Anatomical basis for:

Finding a: ______________________________

____

____

Finding b: ______________________________

____

____

Finding c: ______________________________

____

____

Clinical Case 2

A 38-year-old male patient presented to the emergency department with a history of fall on the right shoulder and neck pain due to road traffic accident. On examination of the patient it, was observed that the patient was unable to move his right hand and fingers (Finding a). He had difficulty flexing his wrist (Finding b). He had hyperextended metacarpophalangeal joints and flexed interphalangeal joints (Finding c). The clinician suspected nerve injury lower trunk of the brachial plexus.

1. What is the root value of the lower trunk of brachial plexus? What is the name of this paralysis?
2. What are the anatomical reasons for Findings a, b and c.

Explanation

1. ______________________________

____

____

2. Anatomical basis for:

Finding a: ______________________________

____

____

Finding b: ______________________________

____

____

Finding c: ______________________________

____

____

PRACTICE FIGURES

(Label the practice figures)

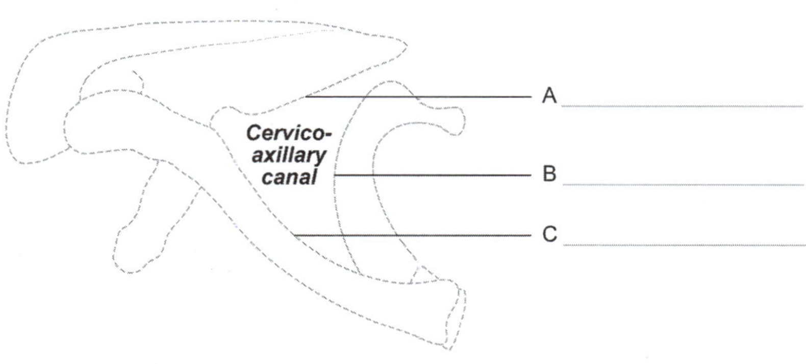

Practice Figure 4.1: Boundaries of apex of axilla or cervicoaxillary canal

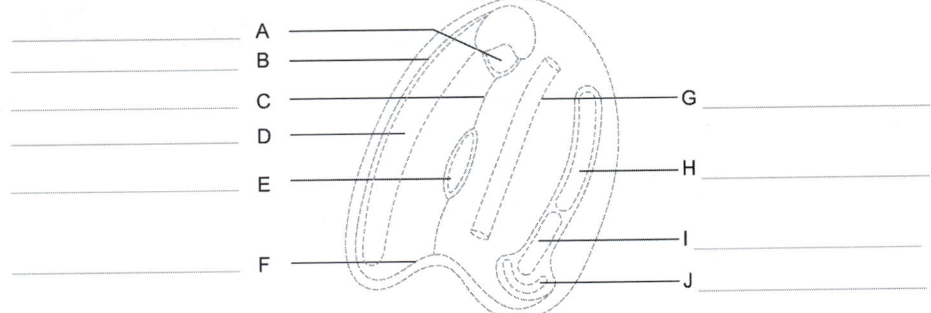

Practice Figure 4.2: Anterior and posterior walls and the base of the axilla with the axillary artery

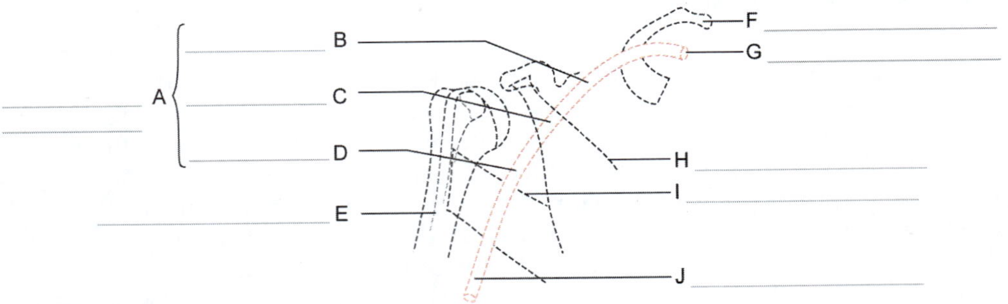

Practice Figure 4.3: The extent and parts of the axillary artery

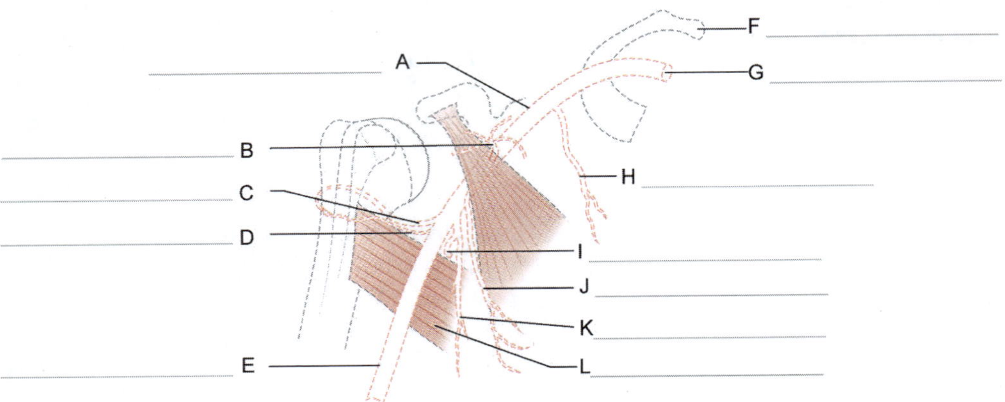

Practice Figure 4.4: The branches of the axillary artery

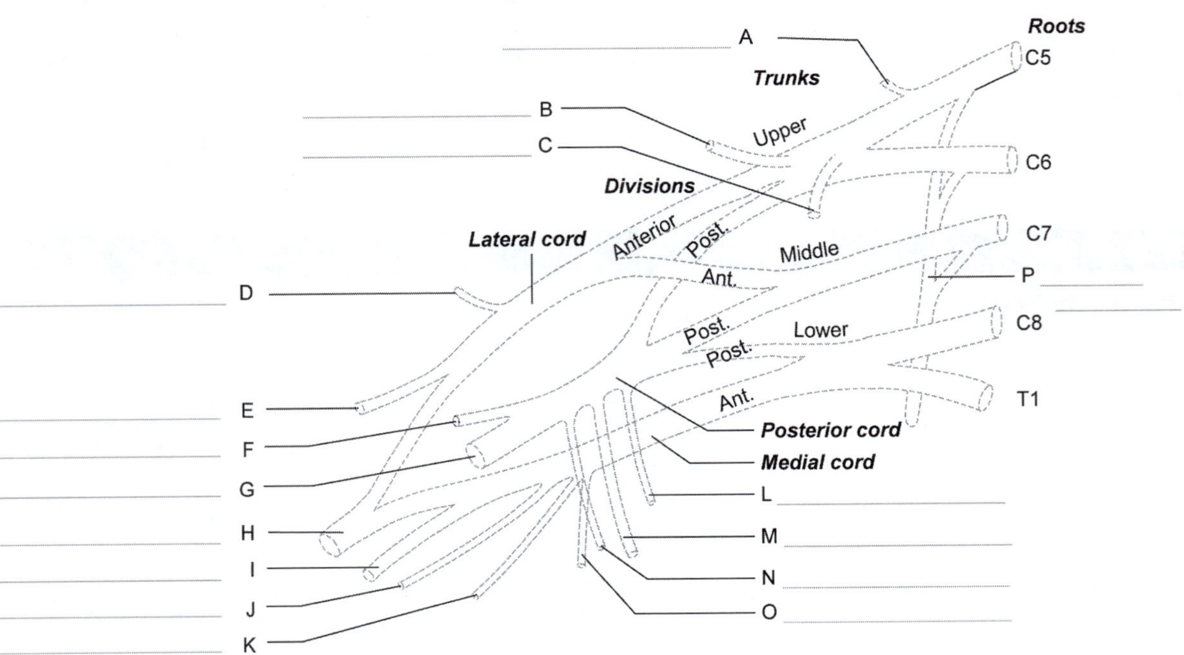

Practice Figure 4.5: The brachial plexus

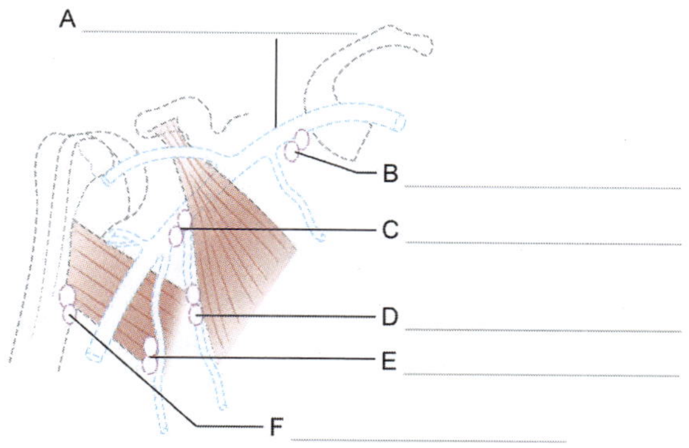

Practice Figure 4.6: The axillary lymph nodes

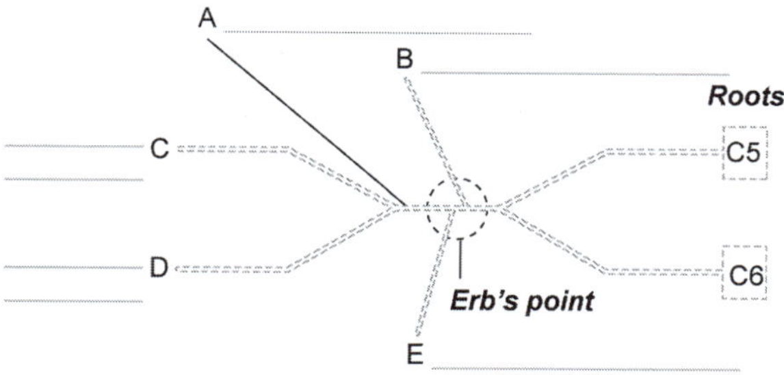

Practice Figure 4.7: Erb's point

MULTIPLE CHOICE QUESTIONS

(Tick the single best correct option)

1. The nerve roots involved the Klumpke's paralysis are:
   a. C5 and C6 b. C6 and C7
   c. C7 and C8 d. C8 and T1
2. The suprascapular nerve arises from ____________.
   a. C5 root b. Upper trunk
   c. Lateral cord d. Posterior cord
3. Lymphatics from the thumb is drained primarily into ____________ group of axillary lymph nodes.
   a. Lateral b. Posterior
   c. Anterior d. Apical
4. Which of the following arteries has an ascending branch that runs in the intertubercular sulcus?
   a. Subscapular artery
   b. Thoracoacromial artery
   c. Anterior circumflex humeral artery
   d. Posterior circumflex humeral artery
5. Damage to which of the following fibres produces Horner's syndrome?
   a. C6 b. C7
   c. C8 d. T1
6. Which of the following is the branch of the second part of the axillary artery?
   a. Subscapular artery
   b. Thoracoacromial artery
   c. Superior thoracic artery
   d. Posterior circumflex humeral artery
7. All of the following are the features of the Klumpke's paralysis, EXCEPT:
   a. Claw hand
   b. Horner's syndrome
   c. Loss of biceps and supinator jerks
   d. Sensory loss along the medial border of forearm and hand
8. The cervicoaxillary canal is bounded by all of the following structures, EXCEPT:
   a. Clavicle
   b. Upper border of scapula
   c. Shaft of humerus
   d. Outer border of the 1st rib
9. Kuntz's nerve is the communicating branch between:
   a. C7 and C8 b. C8 and T1
   c. T1 and T2 d. T2 and T3
10. Which of the following nerves runs on the anterior surface of the subscapularis muscle?
    a. Lower subscapular nerve
    b. Nerve to latissimus dorsi
    c. Upper subscapular nerve
    d. All of the above
11. Identify the nerve marked with X.

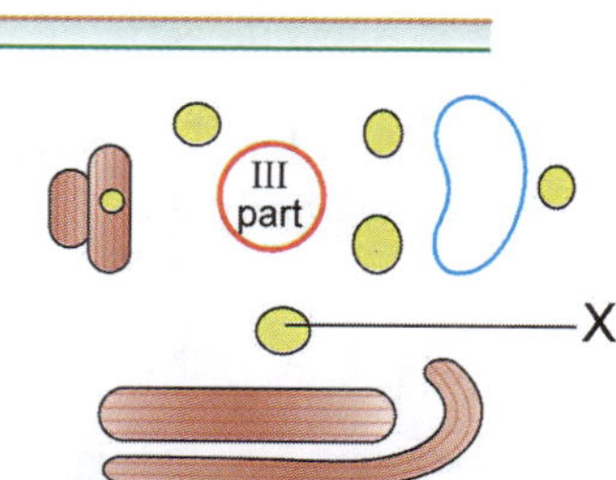

    a. Median nerve b. Radial nerve
    c. Ulnar nerve d. Musculocutaneous nerve
12. Identify the vein marked with X.

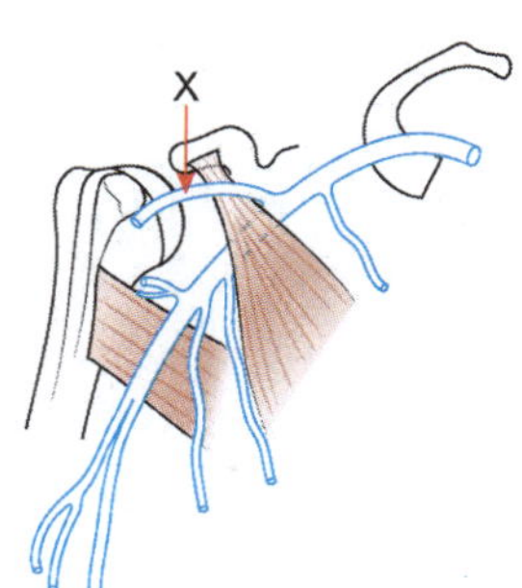

    a. Subclavian vein b. Cephalic vein
    c. Basilic vein d. Brachial vein

QUESTION BANK

(Use separate copy to solve the following questions)

Q 1. Describe the boundaries and content of axilla.

Q 2. Describe the axillary artery under the following headings: Beginning, course and branches.

Q 3. Describe the brachial plexus under the following headings: Formation, branches and applied aspects.

Q 4. Write a short note on:
   a. Axillary lymph nodes
   b. Erb's paralysis
   c. Klumpke's paralysis

Q 5. Enumerate:
   a. Boundaries of axilla
   b. Contents of axilla
   c. Branches of axillary artery
   d. Features of Horner's syndrome
   e. Areas draining into various groups of axillary lymph nodes

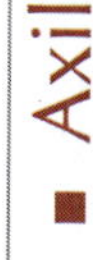

Chapter

5

eSmartQuiz

Back

CLINICOANATOMICAL PROBLEM

Clinical Case 1

A poor young adult male felt multiple nodules in the region of his neck above the clavicle. A lymph node biopsy was advised from right side of his neck. A few days after the biopsy, he was unable to shrug his right shoulder

1. Which muscle was paralysed in this patient?
2. What is the reason for the paralysis?

Explanation

1. ______________________________

____

2. ______________________________

____

____

____

PRACTICE FIGURES

(Label the practice figures)

Practice Figure 5.1: The trapezius muscle and latissimus dorsi

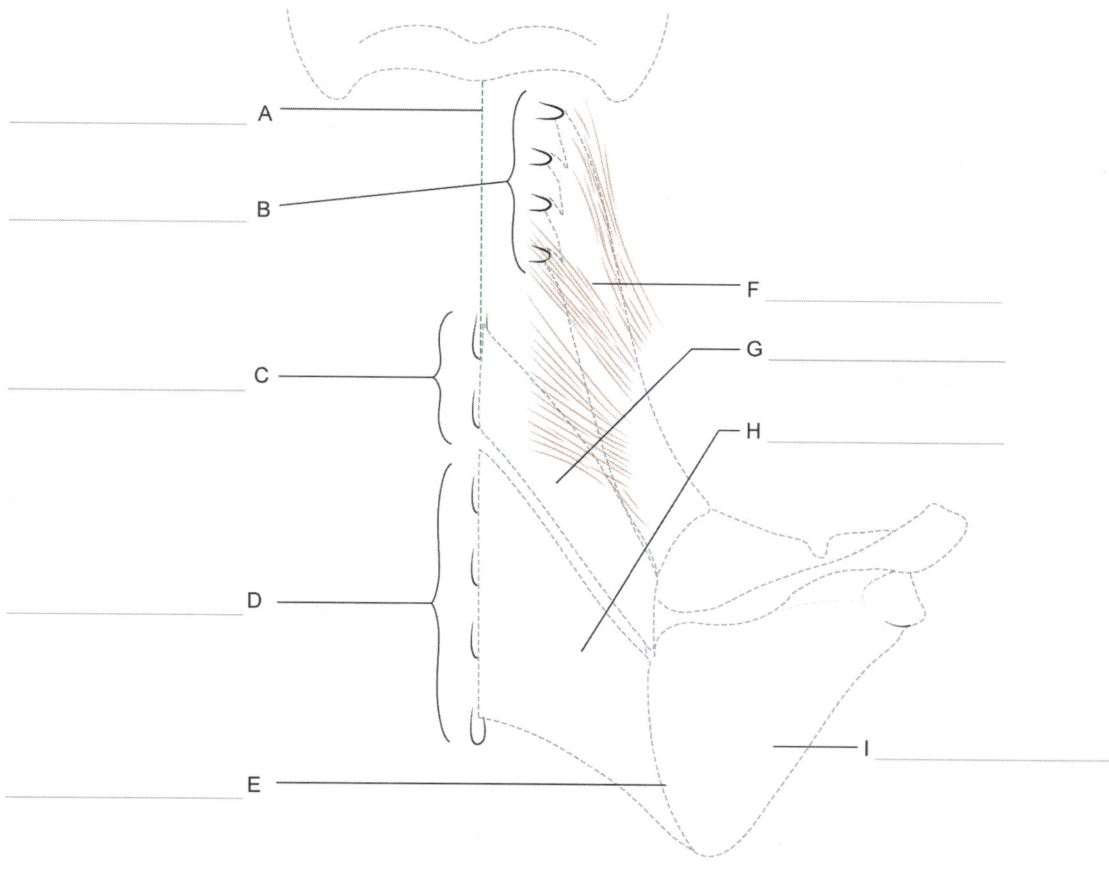

Practice Figure 5.2: The levator scapulae, the rhomboid minor and the rhomboid major muscles

MULTIPLE CHOICE QUESTIONS

(Tick the single best correct option)

1. Paralysis of __________ muscle produces shoulder drop.
   a. Trapezius b. Deltoid
   c. Latissimus dorsi d. Rhomboid major
2. Strangulation of the greater occipital nerve by __________ muscle causes headache from the back of the neck, up over the back of the head.
   a. Levator scapulae b. Latissimus dorsi
   c. Serratus anterior d. Trapezius
3. Which muscle is useful for swimming as well as climbing on the tree?
   a. Teres major b. Deltoid
   c. Trapezius d. Latissimus dorsi
4. What is the clinical importance of the lumbar triangle?
   a. Auscultation of breathing sounds
   b. Petit's hernia
   c. Hematoma formation
   d. Located over the heart
5. Which of the following structures does NOT form the boundary of the triangle of auscultation?
   a. Trapezius b. Levator scapulae
   c. Scapula d. Latissimus dorsi
6. Which of the following structures does NOT form the boundary of the lumbar triangle?
   a. Trapezius
   b. Latissimus dorsi
   c. Iliac crest
   d. External oblique muscle
7. All of the following muscles are supplied by dorsal scapular nerve, EXCEPT:
   a. Rhomboideus minor
   b. Rhomboideus major
   c. Levator scapulae
   d. Trapezius
8. The inferior angle of the scapula lies at the level of __________ vertebra.
   a. T3 b. T5
   c. T7 d. T9
9. Which of the following muscles is inserted in the floor of the bicipital groove?
   a. Trapezius b. Latissimus dorsi
   c. Pectoralis major d. Teres major
10. Which of the following muscles together retract the scapula?
    a. Rhomboid major rhomboid minor
    b. Rhomboid major and levator scapulae
    c. Trapezius and latissimus dorsi
    d. Levator scapulae and latissimus dorsi

QUESTION BANK

(Use separate copy to solve the following questions)

Q 1. Describe trapezius under the following headings:
   a. Origin and insertion
   b. Nerve supply and actions
   c. Structures deep to trapezius
   d. Applied anatomy

Q 2. Write a short note on:
   a. Triangle of auscultation
   b. Lumbar triangle of Petit

Chapter 6

eSmartQuiz

Scapular Region

CLINICOANATOMICAL PROBLEMS

Clinical Case 1

A physician gave an intramuscular injection to a 10-year-old boy in the upper part of the right arm. After one week, a boy came with complaints of pain at the upper part of right arm and difficulty in abduction of the arm. On clinical examination, the sensory loss over the lateral side of the part of arm was noticed.

1. Name the structure damaged due to intramuscular injection.
2. Which muscles are affected in this case?
3. What is the reason for sensory loss?

Explanation

1. ______________________________
2. ______________________________
3. ______________________________

Clinical Case 2

A 20-year-old male cricket player came to the emergency department with complaints of severe pain in the right arm. He fell down on the ground while paying. There were no external signs of the injury. On clinical examination, the weakness in the extension of elbow was noticed along with the numbness in the posterior aspect of forearm. The patient was unable to extend his wrist and fingers. On radiological examination, there was a fracture at the middle of the shaft of the humerus.

1. Name the nerve affected in this patient.
2. Mention the site of lesion in this patient.
3. Why there was a weakness of the extension at the elbow?

Explanation

1. ______________________________
2. ______________________________
3. ______________________________

PRACTICE FIGURES

(Label the practice figures)

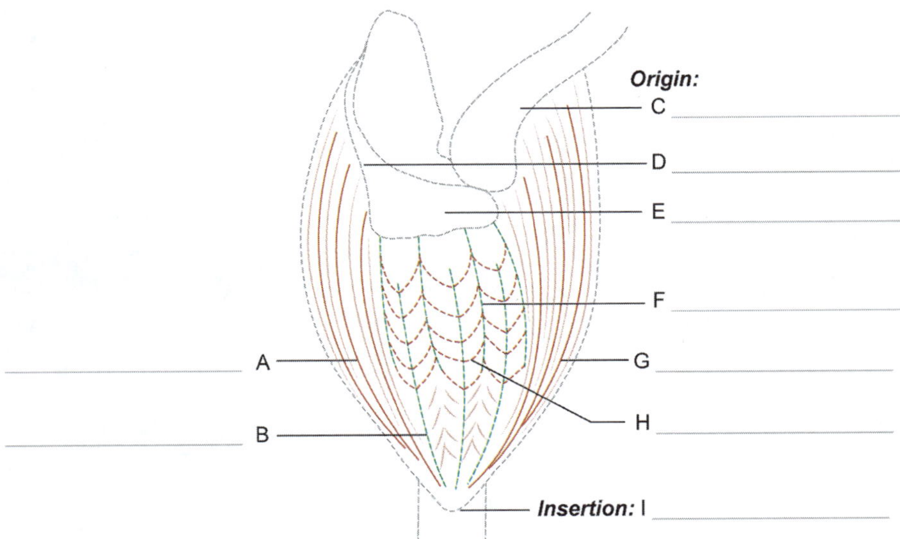

Practice Figure 6.1: Deltoid muscle

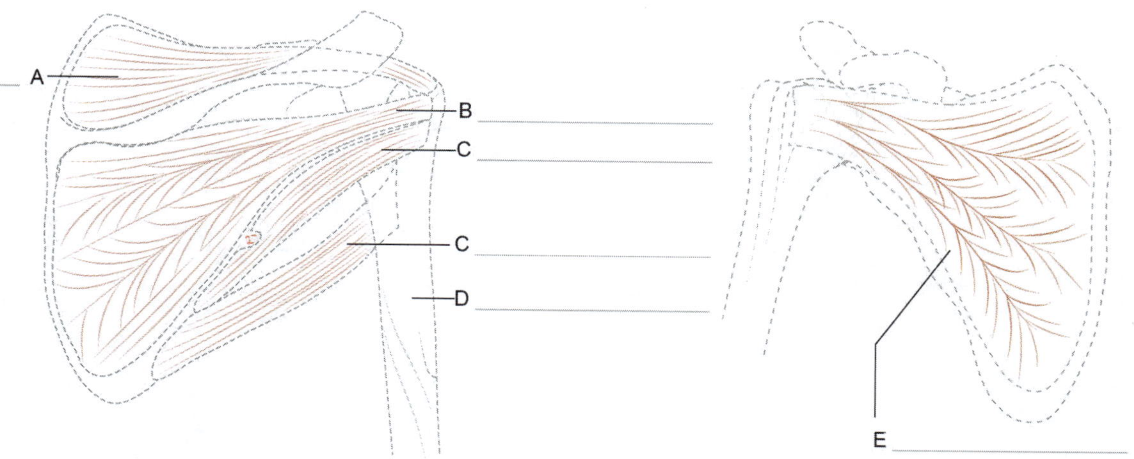

Practice Figure 6.2: Supraspinatus, infraspinatus, teres minor and subscapularis muscles

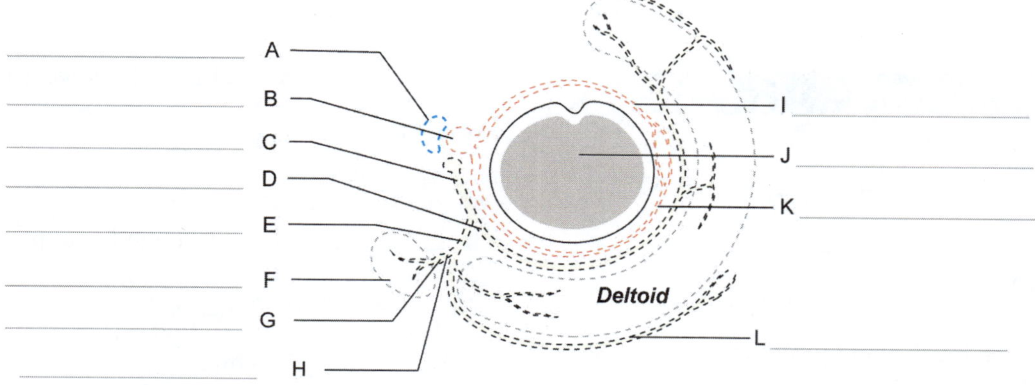

Practice Figure 6.3: Axillary nerve

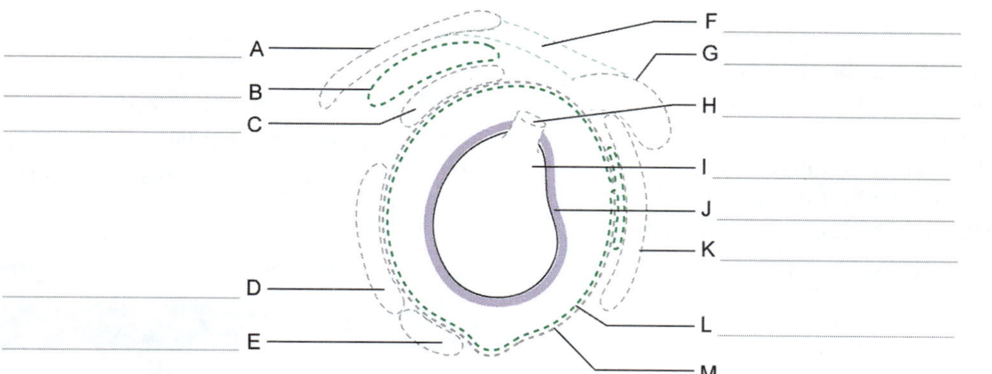

Practice Figure 6.4: Musculotendinous cuff of the shoulder

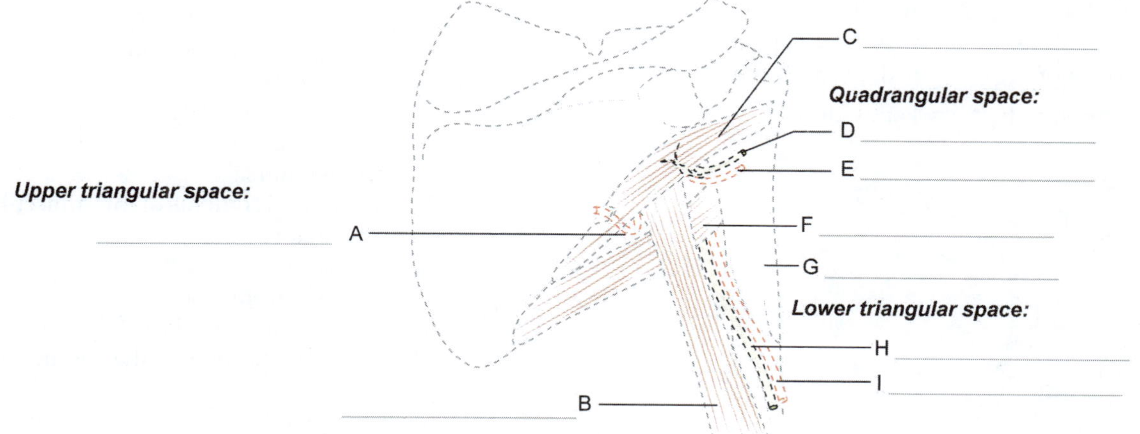

Practice Figure 6.5: The intermuscular spaces in the scapular region

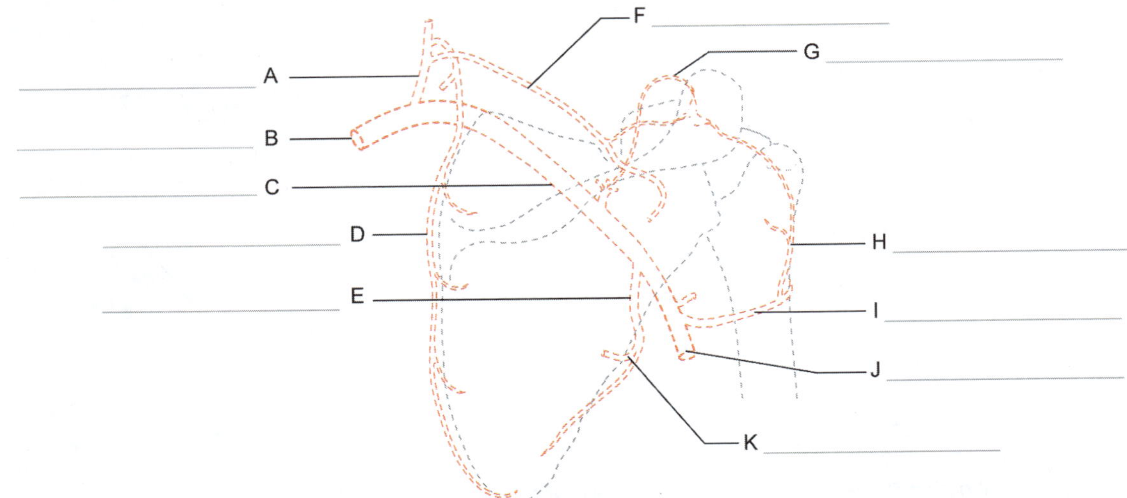

Practice Figure 6.6: Anastomoses around the scapula

MULTIPLE CHOICE QUESTIONS

(Tick the single best correct option)

1. Deltoid muscle is supplied by _______ nerve.
   a. Axillary
   b. Radial
   c. Lower subscapular
   d. Suprascapular
2. ___________ of the deltoid muscle are multipennate.
   a. Clavicular fibres
   b. Acromial fibres
   c. Fibres from spine of scapula
   d. All fibres
3. All of the following may be observed in the paralysis of the deltoid muscle, EXCEPT:
   a. Weakness to abduct the arm
   b. Inability in medial rotation of arm
   c. Loss of rounded contour of shoulder
   d. Sensory loss over the upper half of deltoid
4. Axillary nerve runs along with ___________ artery.
   a. Subscapular
   b. Lateral thoracic
   c. Brachial
   d. Posterior circumflex humeral
5. Which of the following muscles is NOT the component of the rotator cuff of the shoulder?
   a. Subscapularis
   b. Supraspinatus
   c. Teres major
   d. Teres minor
6. Identify the structure marked with X.

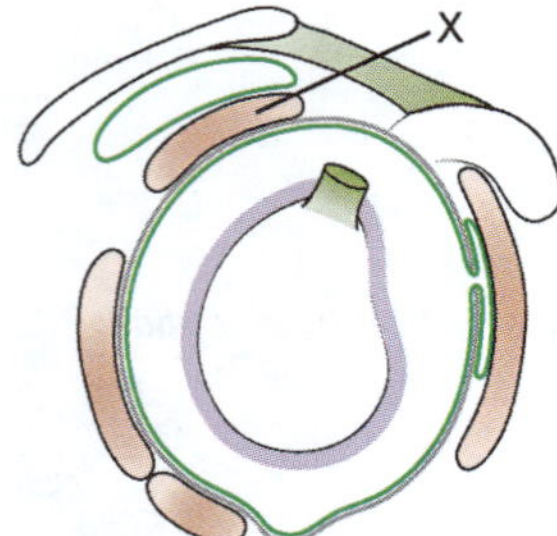

   a. Subscapularis
   b. Supraspinatus
   c. Teres major
   d. Teres minor
7. ___________ is supplied by the lower subscapular nerve.
   a. Teres major
   b. Supraspinatus
   c. Deltoid
   d. Teres minor
8. ___________ passes through the upper triangular intermuscular space.
   a. Axillary nerve
   b. Radial nerve
   c. Profunda brachii artery
   d. Circumflex scapular artery
9. ________ passes through the quadrangular intermuscular space.
   a. Axillary nerve
   b. Radial nerve
   c. Profunda brachii artery
   d. Circumflex scapular artery
10. Regimental-badge anaesthesia is seen in the injury of ___________ nerve.
    a. Radial nerve
    b. Long thoracic nerve
    c. Axillary nerve
    d. Suprascapular nerve

QUESTION BANK

(Use separate copy to solve the following questions)

Q 1. Describe the muscle of the rotator cuff of the shoulder under the following headings:
   a. Origin
   b. Insertion
   c. Nerve supply
   d. Actions
   e. Applied aspects

Q 2. Write a shote note on:
   a. Deltoid muscle
   b. Subacromial bursa
   c. Boundaries and contents of intermuscular spaces of scapular region
   d. Axillary nerve
   e. Anastomosis around scapula

Q 3. Explain anatomical basis of the following:
   a. Intramuscular injections in the middle part of deltoid muscle
   b. Dawbarn's sign
   c. Painful arc syndrome
   d. Regimental-badge anaesthesia

Cutaneous Nerves, Superficial Veins and Lymphatic Drainage

eSmartQuiz

CLINICOANATOMICAL PROBLEMS

Clinical Case 1

A patient had a history of fever since one week. The treating physician asked for blood tests. The intern decided to collect the venous blood sample from the upper limb.

1. Which vein is commonly preferred for blood sample collection in the upper limb?
2. Why this vein was selected?
3. How does one make the veins prominent?

Explanation

1. ______________________
2. ______________________
3. ______________________

Clinical Case 2

A 30-year-old farmer noticed swelling and tenderness in his left armpit. He recently had a minor cut on his left thumb while working in the farm. Despite cleaning and bandaging the wound, he noticed some redness and swelling around the area in the following days. During the physical examination, the physician noticed the enlarged and tender lymph nodes in the left axilla and redness and warmth over the affected area of the thumb.

1. Which group of the axillary lymph nodes primarily drain the lymphatics from the thumb?
2. What is the location of these lymph nodes?

Explanation

1. ______________________
2. ______________________

PRACTICE FIGURES

(Label the practice figures)

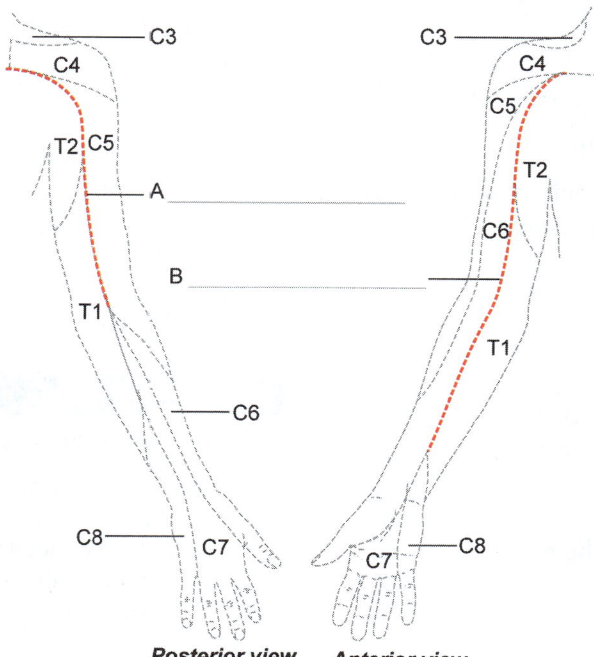

Practice Figure 7.1: Dermatomes of upper limb

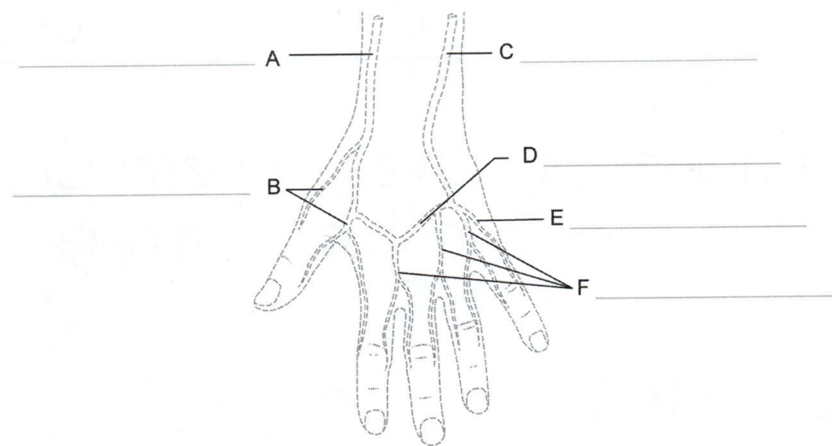

Practice Figure 7.2: Dorsal venous arch

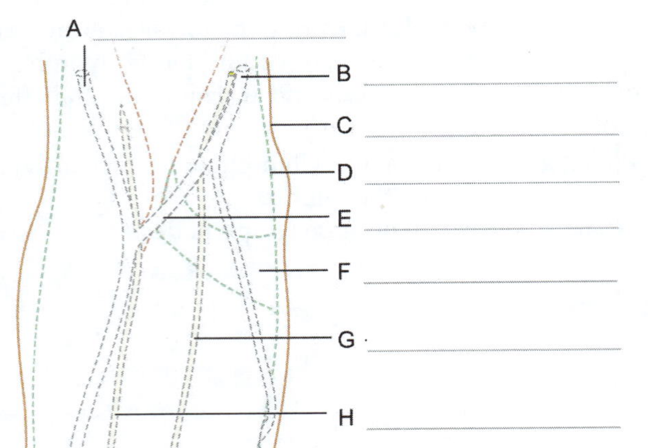

Practice Figure 7.3: Median cubital vein and roof of cubital fossa

MULTIPLE CHOICE QUESTIONS

(Tick the single best correct option)

1. The lateral cutaneous nerve of forearm is a continuation of ____________ nerve.
   a. Axillary b. Median
   c. Radial d. Musculocutaneous
2. Supraclavicular nerve supplies the skin of the pectoral region up to the level of ____________ rib.
   a. First b. Second
   c. Third d. Fourth
3. Which of the following veins is stabilised by the perforator passing through the bicipital aponeurosis?
   a. Cephalic
   b. Basilic
   c. Median cubital
   d. Median vein of the forearm
4. Lymph shed line on the ____________ of the arm.
   a. Lateral side b. Medial side
   c. Anterior aspect d. Posterior aspect
5. Spinal segments T1–T6 lie opposite:
   a. Spines of 1–4 thoracic vertebrae
   b. Spines of 1–6 thoracic vertebrae
   c. Spines of 2–7 thoracic spines
   d. Spines of 2–8 thoracic spines
6. The ____________ dermatome corresponds to the little finger.
   a. C6 b. C7
   c. C8 d. T1
7. ____________ is the most commonly used vein for intravenous injections.
   a. Cephalic vein
   b. Basilic vein
   c. Median cubital vein
   d. Median vein of the forearm
8. Skin over the thenar eminence is supplied by ________ nerve.
   a. Ulnar b. Median
   c. Radial d. Anterior interosseous
9. Intercostobrachial nerve is the lateral cutaneous branch of ____________ intercostal nerve.
   a. First b. Second
   c. Third d. Fourth
10. The posterior cutaneous nerve of forearm is a branch of ____________ nerve.
    a. Axillary b. Median
    c. Radial d. Musculocutaneous
11. The medial end of the dorsal venous arch of the hand continues as:
    a. Cephalic
    b. Basilic
    c. Median cubital
    d. Median vein of the forearm
12. The ______________ dermatome corresponds to the thumb.
    a. C6 b. C7
    c. C8 d. T1

QUESTION BANK

(Use separate copy to solve the following questions)

Q 1. Write a short note on:
   a. Cutaneous nerve supply of palm
   b. Dorsal venous arch of hand
   c. Median cubital vein
   d. Axillary lymph nodes

Chapter

8

eSmartQuiz

Arm

CLINICOANATOMICAL PROBLEM

Clinical Case 1

A 25-year-old construction worker was involved in a workplace accident where he fell from a ladder and landed on his outstretched right arm. Following the accident, he experienced severe pain and weakness in his right upper limb. On clinical examination, clinician observed that the patient had difficulty in flexing his right elbow (Finding a) and a sensory loss along the lateral aspect of the forearm (Finding b).

1. Which nerve in this patient was damaged?
2. What are the anatomical reasons for Findings a and b.

Explanation

1. ______________________________

2. Anatomical basis for:

Finding a: ______________________________

Finding b: ______________________________

PRACTICE FIGURES

(Label the practice figures)

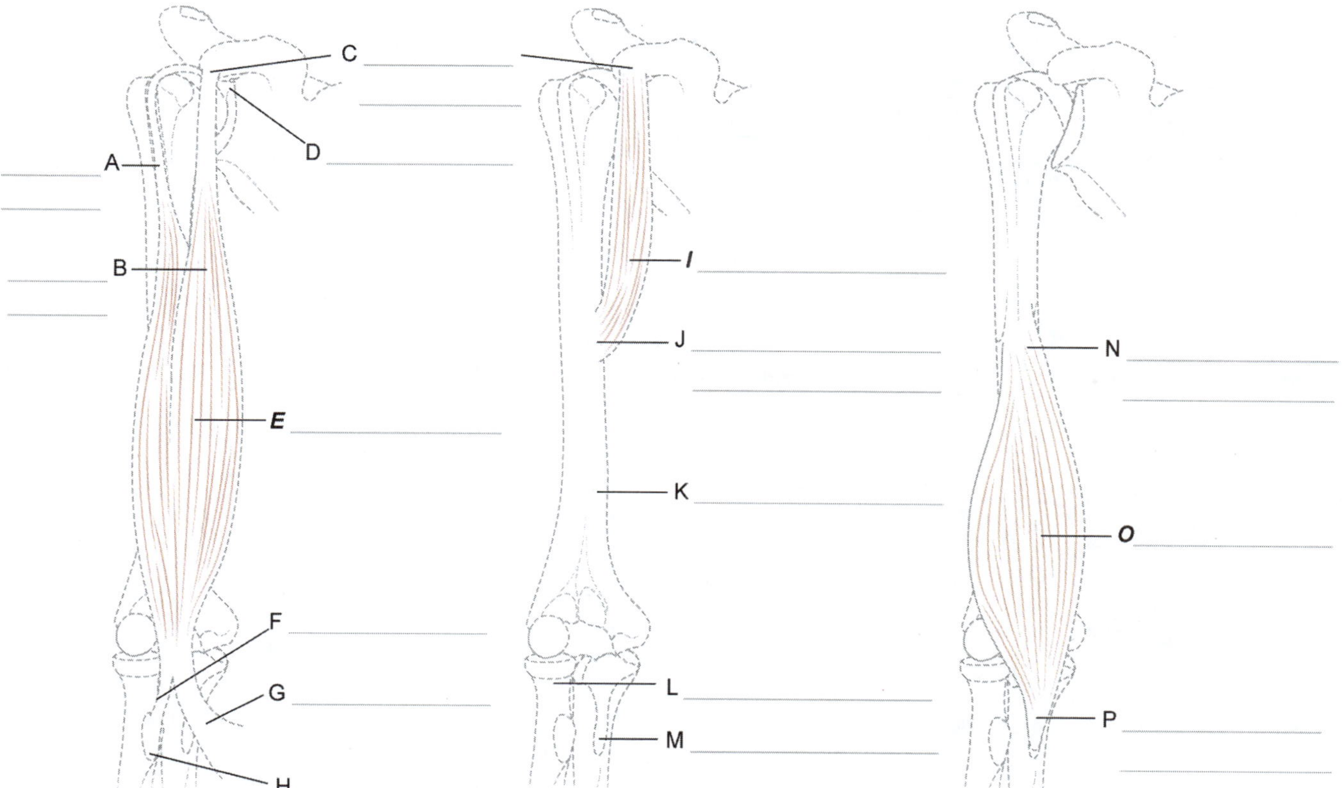

Practice Figure 8.1: Biceps brachii, coracobrachialis and brachialis muscles

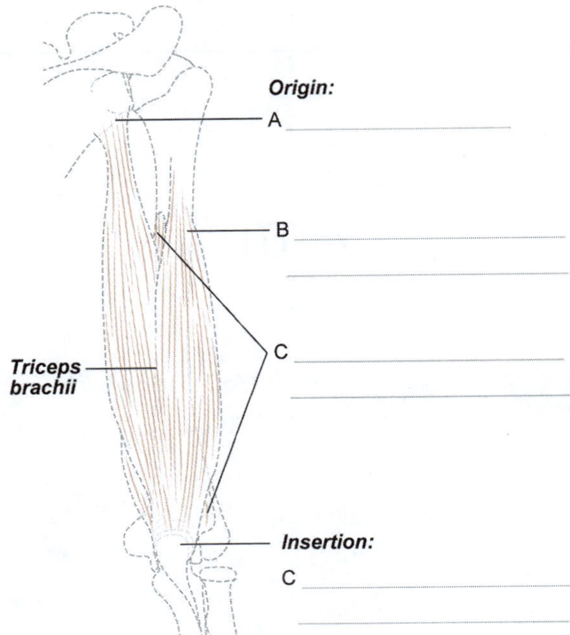

Practice Figure 8.2: Triceps brachii muscle

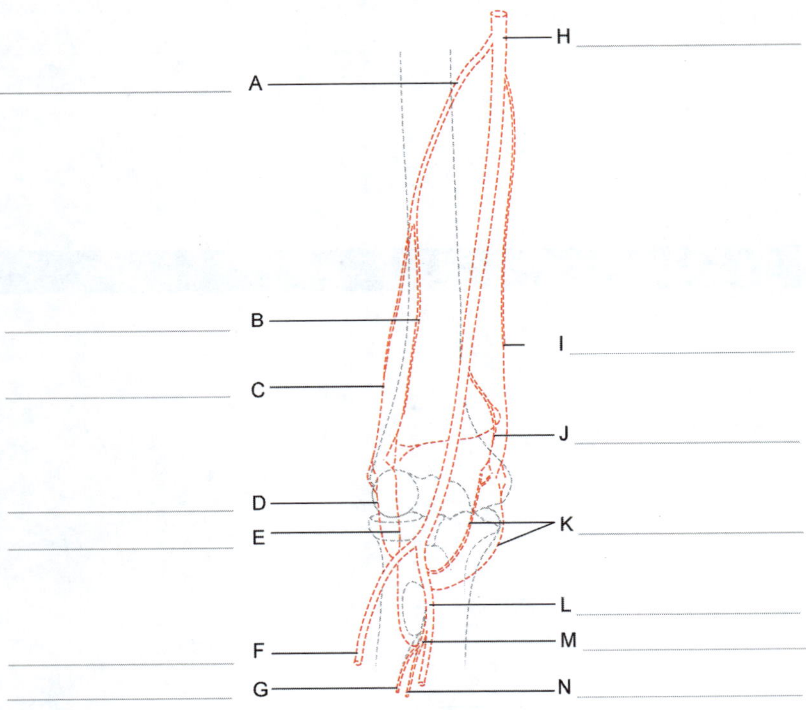

Practice Figure 8.3: Anastomosis around elbow

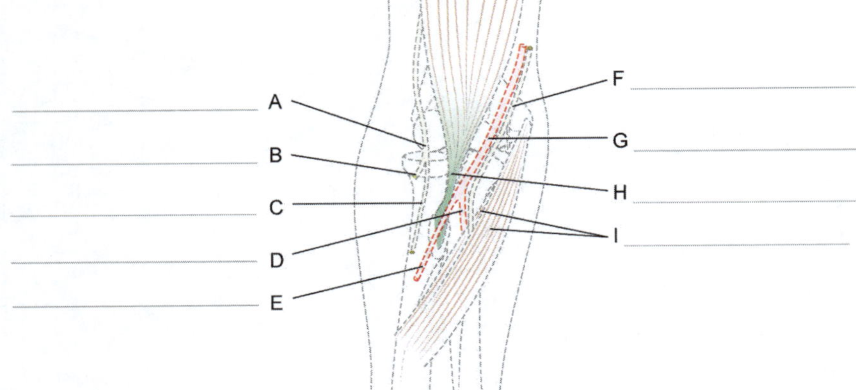

Practice Figure 8.4: Contents of right cubital fossa

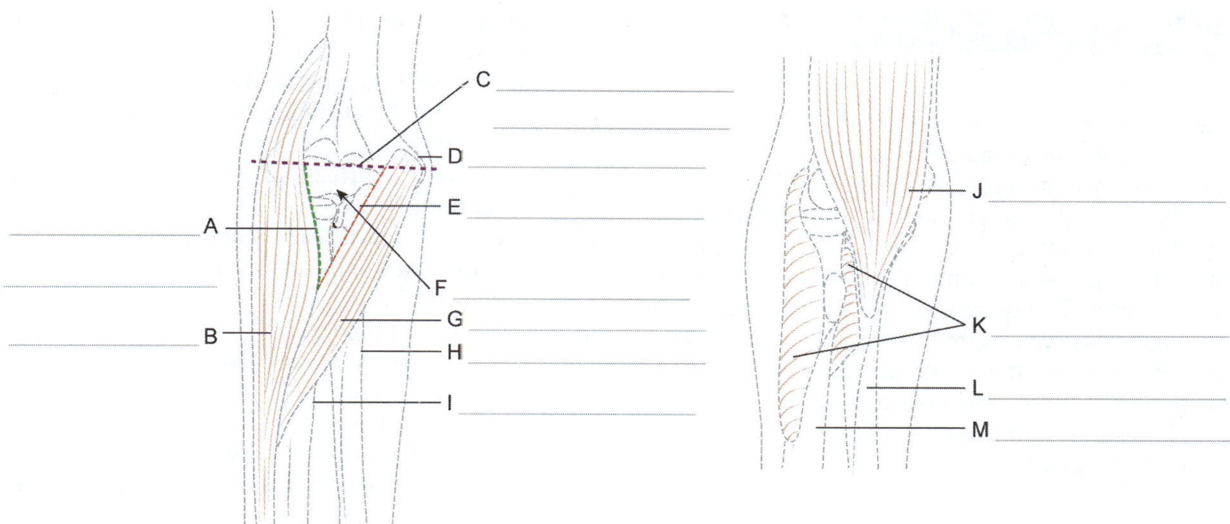

Practice Figure 8.5: Boundaries and floor of cubital fossa

MULTIPLE CHOICE QUESTIONS

(Tick the single best correct option)

1. Which of the following nerves passes through the spiral groove of the humerus?
   a. Ulnar b. Median
   c. Radial d. Axillary
2. To determine if biceps tendon is stable in bicipital groove, the test was performed. During this test, the patient's elbow is flexed to 90 degrees, and the forearm is pronated against resistance while the examiner simultaneously palpates the bicipital groove and monitors for any subluxation or popping of the biceps tendon. What is the name of this test?
   a. Yergason test b. Drop arm test
   c. Ludington's test d. O'Brien's test
3. In case of an injury to the musculocutaneous nerve, which of the following muscles can produce flexion at the elbow?
   a. Brachialis b. Brachioradialis
   c. Coracobrachialis d. Biceps brachii
4. Which of the following muscles has a dual nerve supply?
   a. Biceps brachii b. Brachialis
   c. Triceps brachii d. Brachioradialis
5. Which of the following muscles represents the medial compartment of arm?
   a. Biceps brachii b. Brachialis
   c. Triceps brachii d. Coracobrachialis
6. Which of the following is the Casser's perforated muscle?
   a. Biceps brachii
   b. Brachialis
   c. Triceps brachii
   d. Coracobrachialis
7. Which of the following is not observed in a case of damage to the musculocutaneous nerve?
   a. Loss of biceps tendon reflex
   b. Weakness of lateral rotation of arm
   c. Weakness of flexion of elbow
   d. Loss of cutaneous sensation along the lateral aspect of forearm
8. All of the following are branches of brachial artery, EXCEPT:
   a. Profunda brachii artery
   b. Nutrient artery of humerus
   c. Radial collateral artery
   d. Inferior ulnar collateral artery
9. Which of the following parts of the triceps brachii are supplied by the radial nerve before it enters the radial groove?
   a. Long and medial head
   b. Long and lateral head
   c. Medial and lateral heads
   d. Entire muscle
10. Identify the structure marked with X.

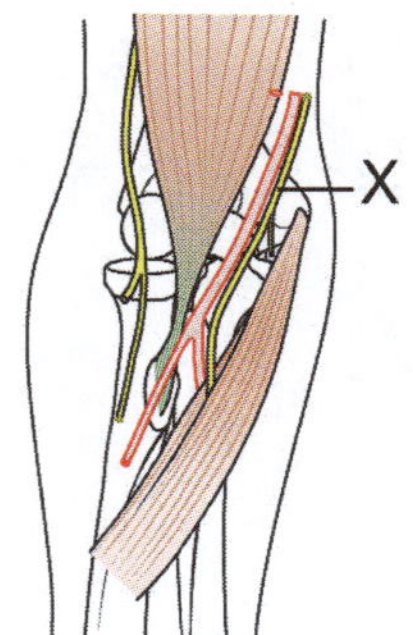

   a. Median nerve
   b. Radial nerve
   c. Ulnar nerve
   d. Medial cutaneous nerve of forearm
11. Identify the structure marked with X.

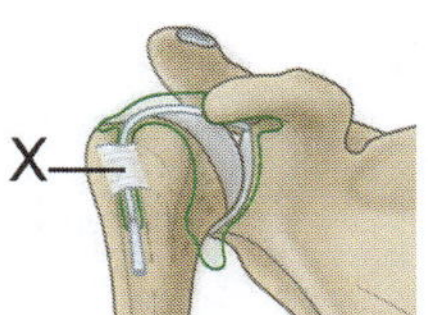

   a. Coracohumeral ligament
   b. Coracoacromial ligament
   c. Transverse humeral ligament
   d. Glenohumeral ligament

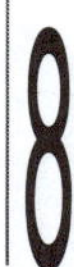

QUESTION BANK

(Use separate copy to solve the following questions)

Q 1. A 35-year-old man was involved in a motorcycle accident where he sustained a traumatic injury to his right upper limb. Upon evaluation at the emergency department, it was noted that the patient had experienced significant impact on the lateral aspect of his arm during the accident. On physical examination, the doctor observed that the patient had difficulty extending his right wrist and fingers. Sensory examination revealed numbness and tingling along the dorsal aspect of his hand and fingers. Furthermore, weakness in supination and radial deviation of the wrist was noted. The doctor diagnosed it as a case of radial nerve injury.

Based on this clinical scenario answer the following question:

a. Explain the course and relations of the radial nerve.
b. Explain the site where the radial nerve was damaged in this case.
c. Enlist the effects of the radial nerve injuries at various sites.

Q 2. Describe the brachial artery under the following headings: Beginning, terminations, course, relations, branches and applied aspects.

Q 3. Write a short note on:

a. Anastomosis around the elbow
b. Biceps brachii
c. Coracobrachialis
d. Musculocutaneous nerve
e. Injury to the radial nerve in the spiral groove

eSmartQuiz

Forearm and Hand

CLINICOANATOMICAL PROBLEMS

Clinical Case 1

A 22-year-old tennis player presented to her physician with complaints of pain and tenderness on the outer aspect of her right elbow. She reported that the pain began gradually a few weeks ago and has progressively worsened, especially during and after playing tennis. She mentioned that she often uses her right arm for repetitive backhand strokes during her tennis matches. On clinical examination, the physician observed localized tenderness and swelling over the lateral epicondyle of patient's right elbow. Palpation of the area elicited pain, particularly when she performed resisted wrist extension or gripping activities. The physician diagnosed her with tennis elbow.

1. Why does pain occur over lateral epicondyle during tennis games?
2. Which other games can lead to tennis elbow?

Explanation

1. ______________________________

2. ______________________________

Clinical Case 2

A 45-year-old office worker presented to her physician with complaints of numbness, tingling and pain in her right hand and fingers, particularly in the thumb, index and middle fingers. She reported that the symptoms began gradually a few months ago and have progressively worsened, especially at night and during activities that involve repetitive wrist movements, such as typing on the computer keyboard. On clinical examination, the physician noted that the patient had decreased sensation along affected area. Tapping in the middle part of the wrist elicited tingling sensations. The physician diagnosed the patient with carpal tunnel syndrome.

1. Which nerve is involved in the carpal tunnel syndrome?
2. Which movements produced carpal tunnel syndrome in this case?
3. What is the name of the test that elicits the tingling sensation at the wrist?

Explanation

1. ______________________________
2. ______________________________
3. ______________________________

PRACTICE FIGURES

(Label the practice figures)

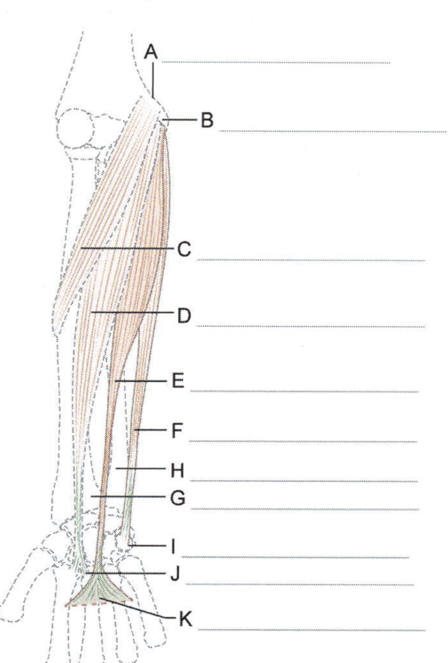

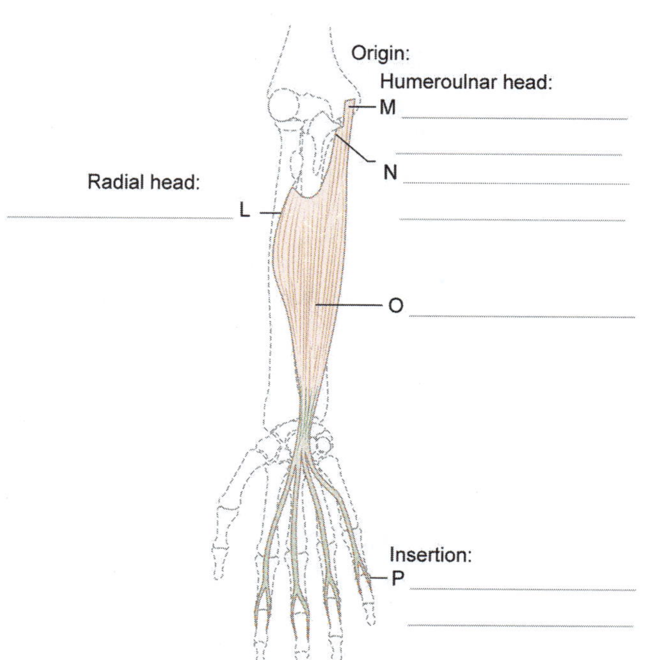

Practice Figure 9.1: Superficial muscles of forearm

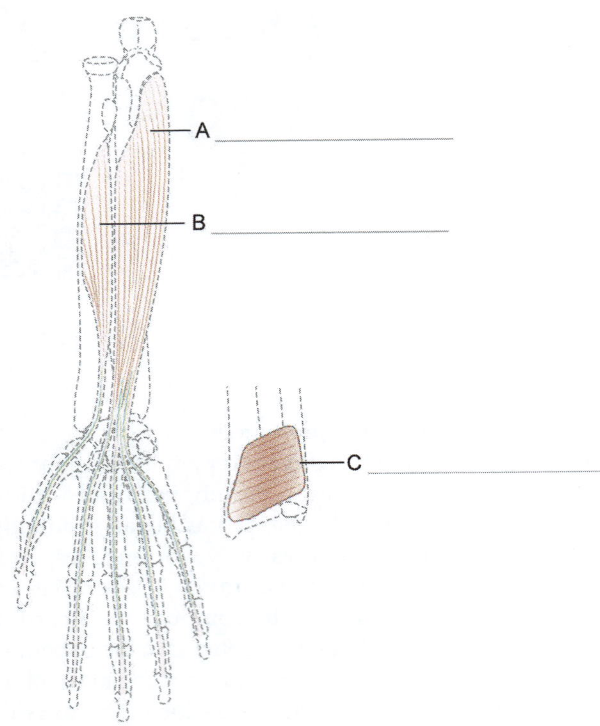

Practice Figure 9.2: Deep muscles of forearm

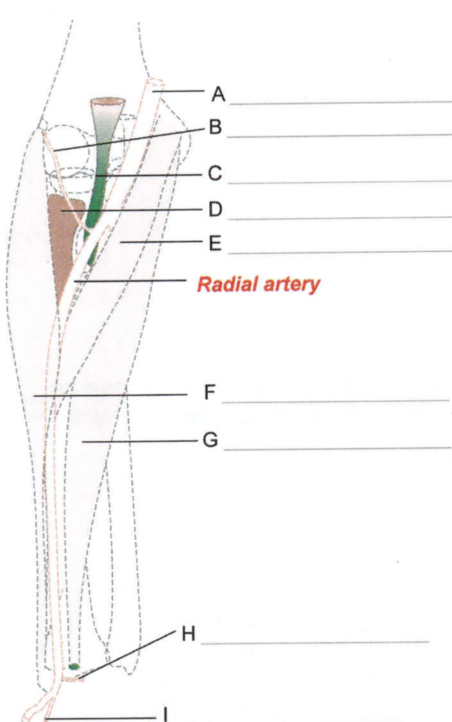

Practice Figure 9.3: Relations of radial artery

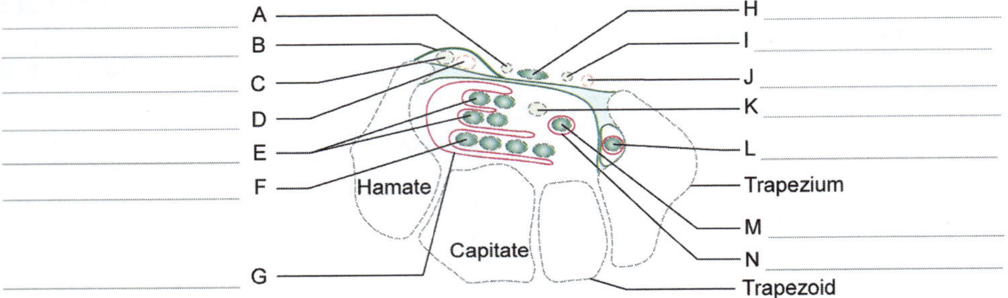

Practice Figure 9.4: Relations of flexor retinaculum

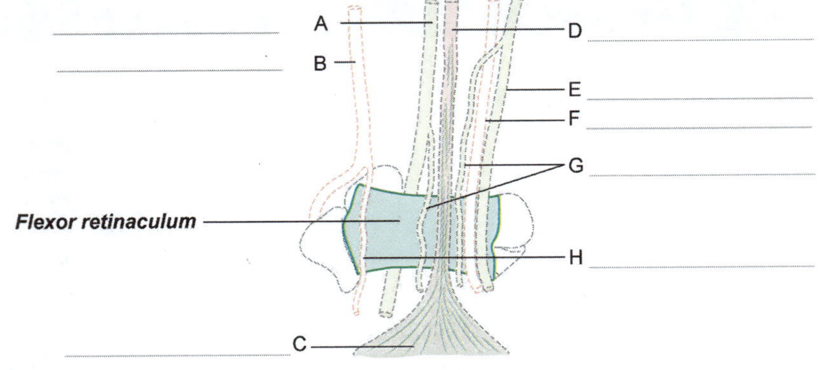

Practice Figure 9.5: Superficial relations of flexor retinaculum

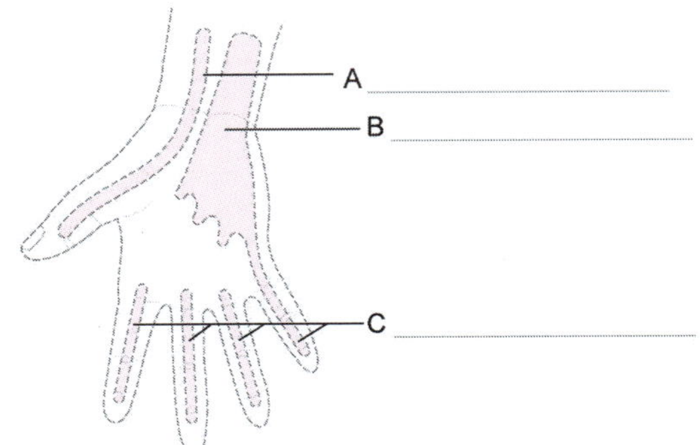

Practice Figure 9.6: Synovial sheaths of the flexor tendons of hand

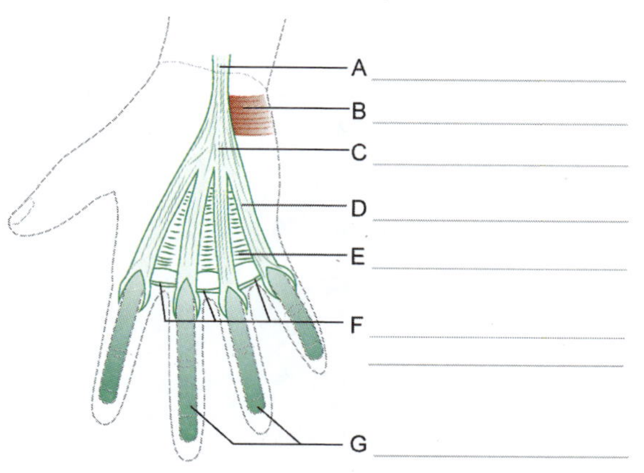

Practice Figure 9.7: Palmar aponeurosis

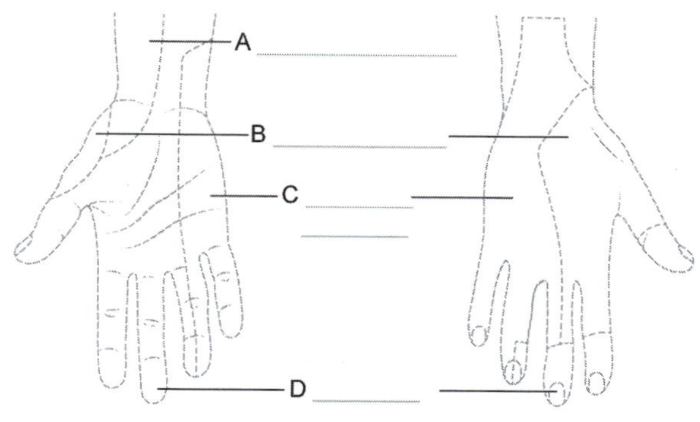

Practice Figure 9.8: Cutaneous innervation of palm and dorsum of hand

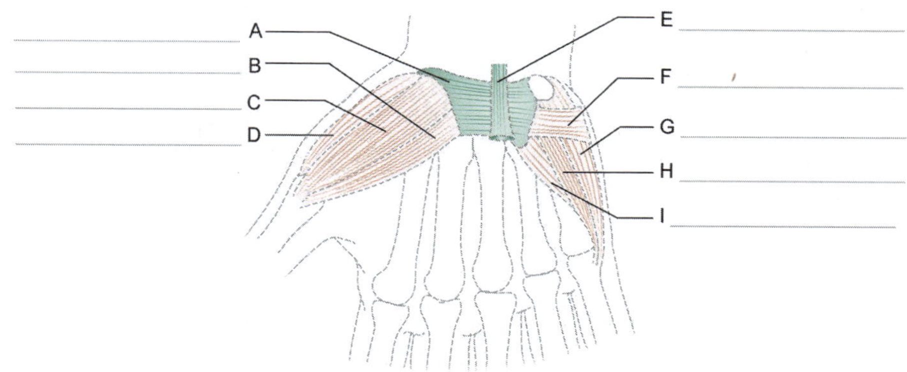

Practice Figure 9.9: Thenar and hypothenar muscles

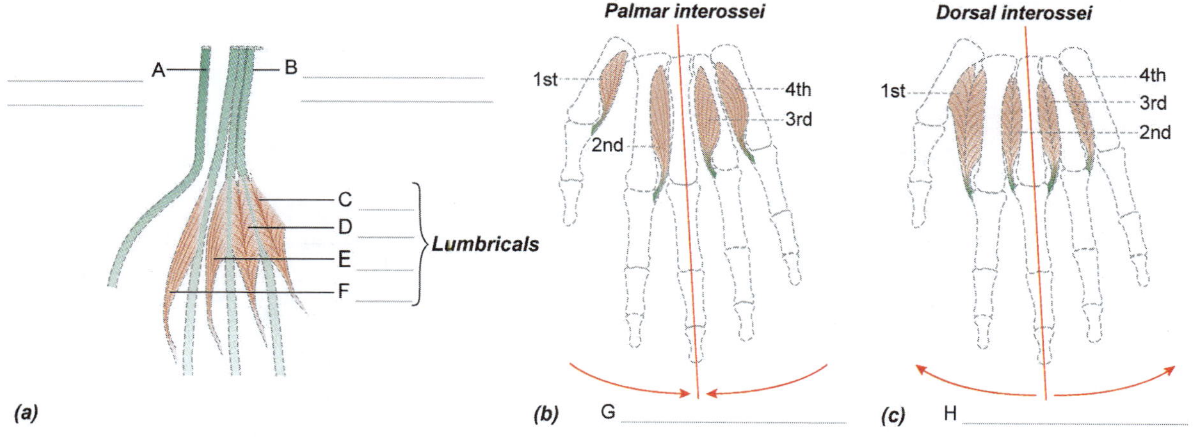

Practice Figure 9.10: Lumbricals and interossei muscles

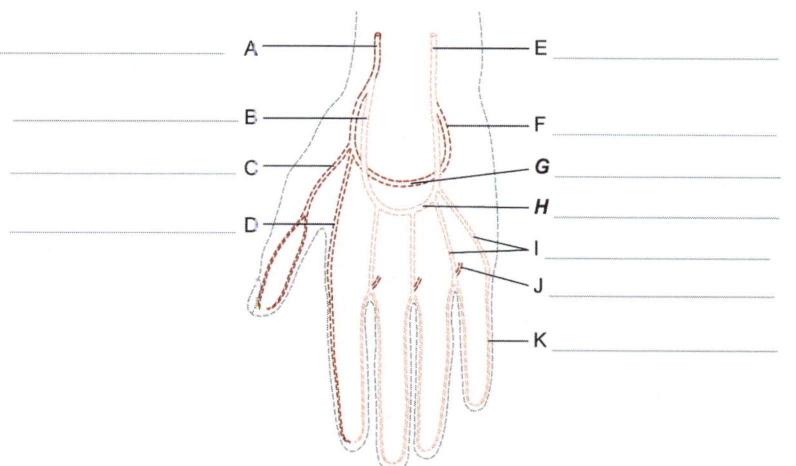

Practice Figure 9.11: The superficial and deep palmar arches

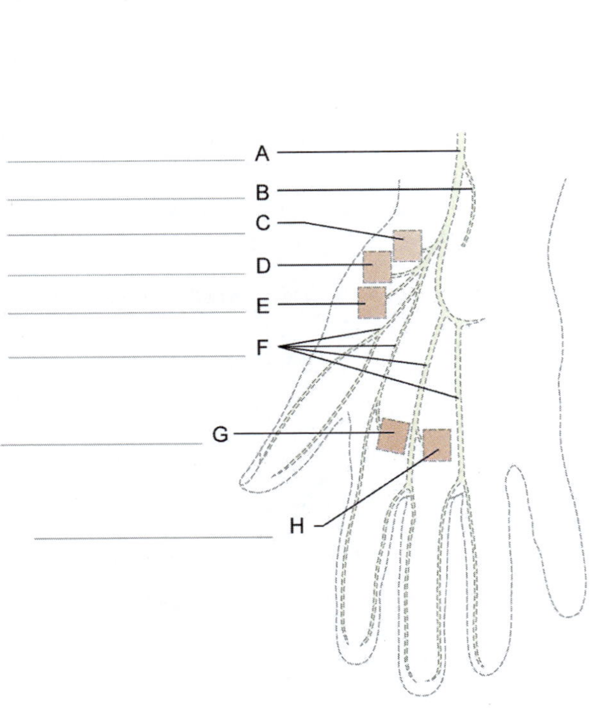

Practice Figure 9.12: Distribution of the median nerve in the hand

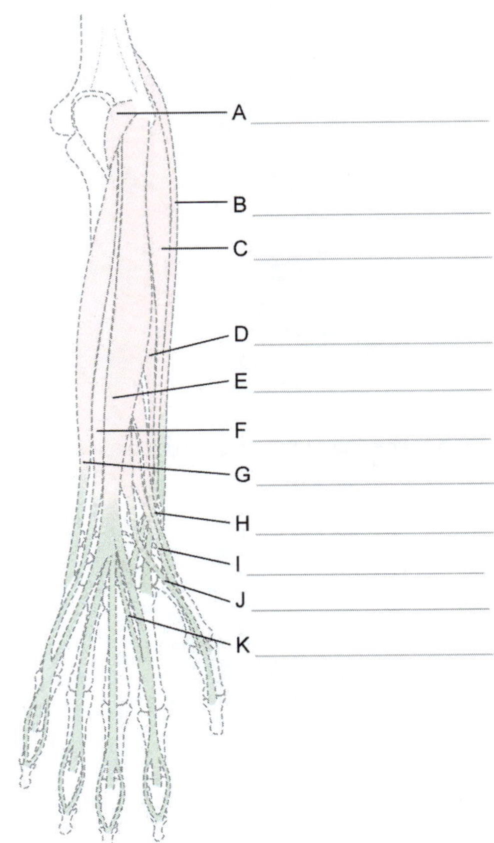

Practice Figure 9.13: Muscles of posterior compartment of forearm

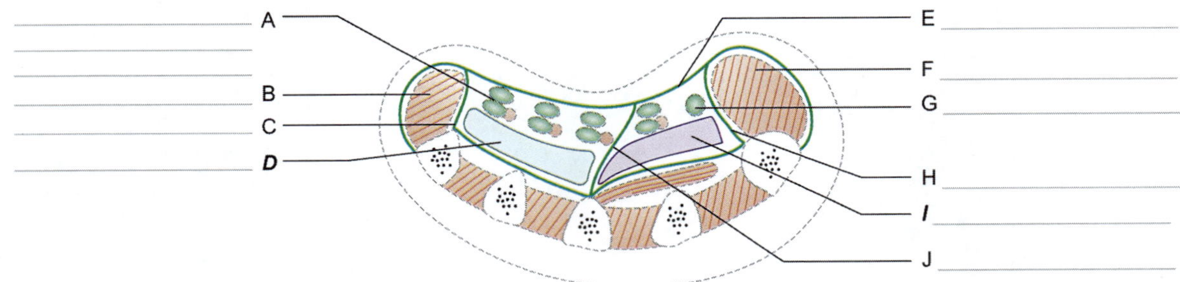

Practice Figure 9.14: Thenar and hypothenar space

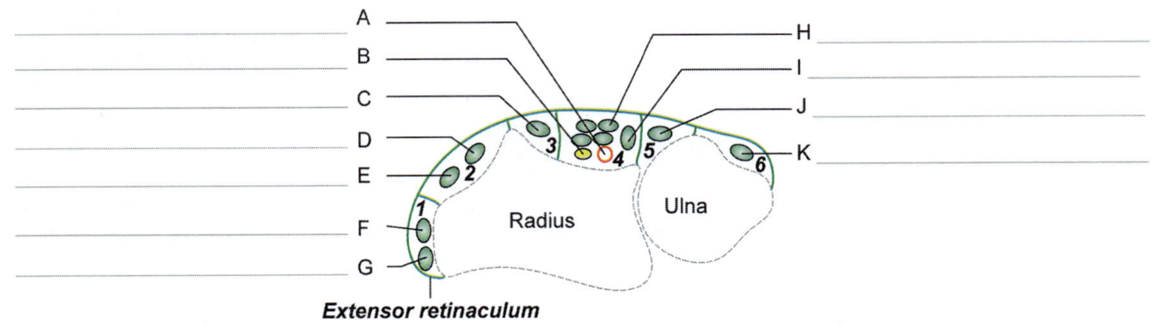

Practice Figure 9.15: Extensor retinaculum

MULTIPLE CHOICE QUESTIONS

(Tick the single best correct option)

1. Identify the structure marked with X.

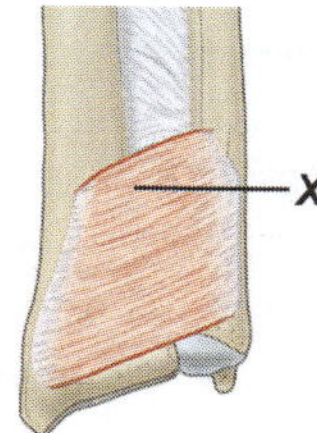

a. Pronator teres
b. Brachioradialis
c. Pronator quadratus
d. Flexor pollicis longus

2. Identify the tendon marked with X which is useful during palpation of the radial artery.

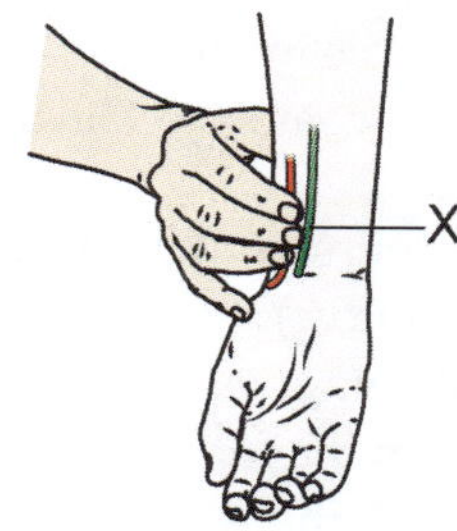

a. Flexor digitorum superficialis
b. Brachioradialis
c. Flexor carpi radialis
d. Flexor pollicis longus

3. Which of the following structures passes through the tunnel marked with X?

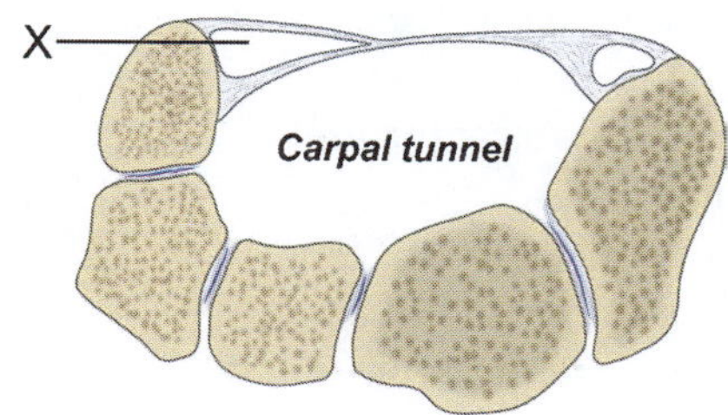

a. Ulnar artery
b. Median nerve
c. Tendon of flexor carpi radialis
d. Redial artery

4. Which structure is affected in the condition shown in the following figure?

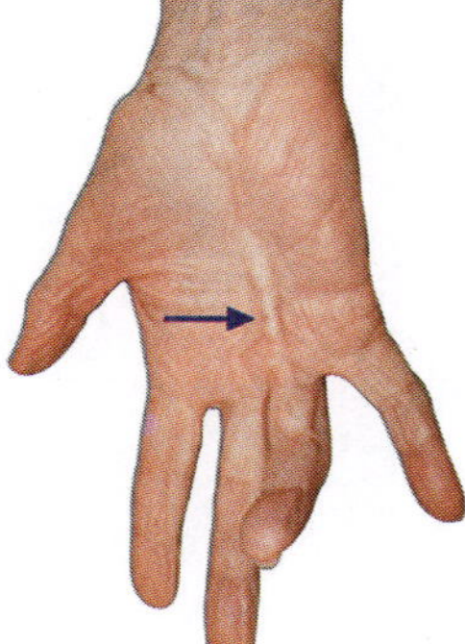

a. Palmar aponeurosis
b. Ulnar bursa
c. Tendons of flexor digitorum superficialis
d. Ulnar nerve

5. Identify the structure marked with X.

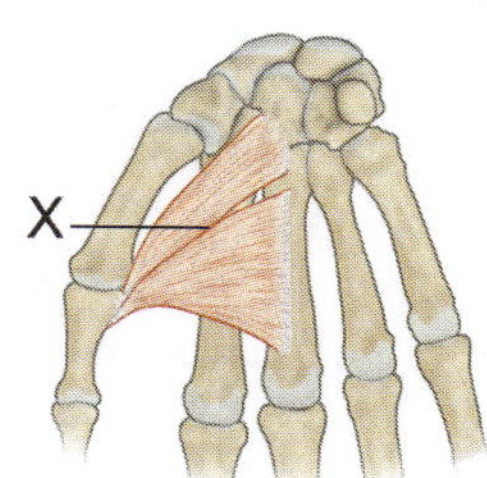

a. Abductor pollicis brevis
b. Flexor pollicis brevis
c. Opponens pollicis
d. Adductor pollicis

6. Which of the following muscles is tested in the following clinical test?

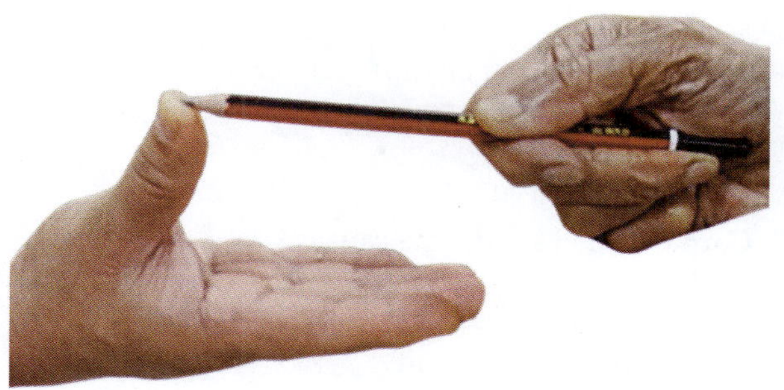

a. Abductor pollicis brevis
b. Flexor pollicis brevis
c. Opponens pollicis
d. Adductor pollicis

7. Identify the structure marked with X.

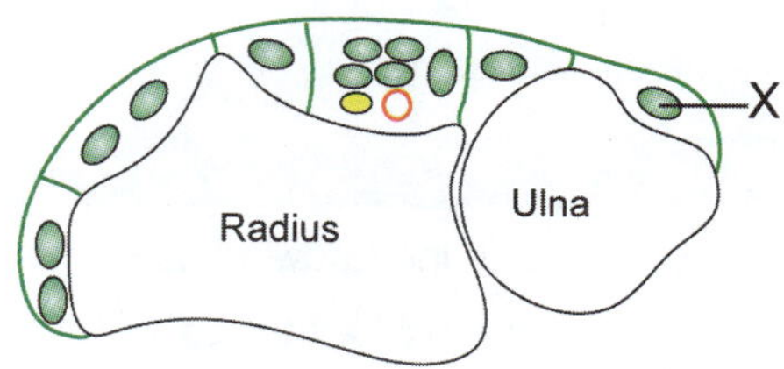

a. Extensor carpi ulnaris
b. Extensor indicis
c. Extensor digitorum
d. Extensor pollicis longus

8. Name the nerve tested in the following clinical test.

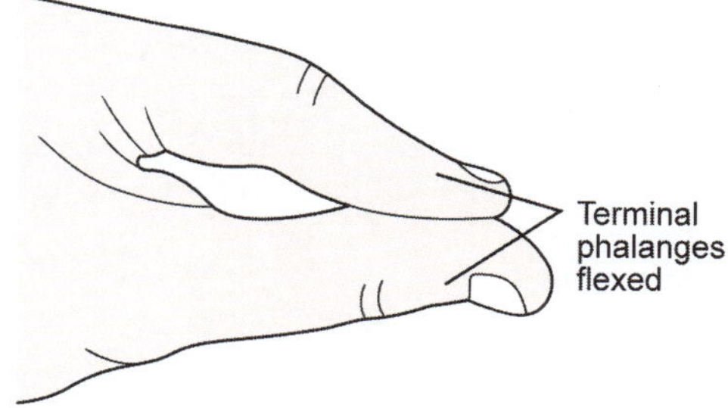

a. Posterior interosseous nerve
b. Superficial branch of radial nerve
c. Deep branch of ulnar nerve
d. Anterior interosseous nerve

9. Interossei inserted into middle finger:
a. Second palmar
b. Second dorsal
c. Third palmar
d. Fourth dorsal

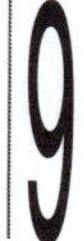

10. Claw hand occurs due to paralysis of ________ muscles.
    a. Palmar interossei
    b. Lumbricals
    c. Flexor digitorum profundus
    d. Flexor digitorum superficialis
11. The ________ passes through the anatomical snuff box.
    a. Superficial branch of radial nerve
    b. Radial artery
    c. Cephalic vein
    d. Tendon of flexor pollicis longus
12. All of the following structures are supplied by anterior interosseous nerve, EXCEPT:
    a. Flexor pollicis longus
    b. Lateral half of flexor digitorum profundus
    c. Pronator teres
    d. Wrist joint
13. Meralgia paraesthetica is caused by injury to:
    a. Superficial branch of radial nerve
    b. Anterior interosseous nerve
    c. Ulnar nerve
    d. Axillary nerve
14. Carpal tunnel syndrome causes ________.
    a. Wrist drop
    b. Claw hand
    c. Waiter's tip deformity
    d. Ape thumb deformity
15. In case of injury to the ________ nerve, if a patient tries to make a fist, the index and middle fingers may remain partially extended.
    a. Ulnar nerve
    b. Radial nerve
    c. Median nerve
    d. Musculocutaneous nerve

QUESTION BANK

(Use separate copy to solve the following questions)

Q 1. A 35-year-old male was admitted to the department of plastic, hand and reconstructive surgery due to persistent loss of sensation of the thenar area and a soft tissue laceration of the palmar wrist following a road accident a week before. The doctor diagnosed it is a case of median nerve injury. Discuss the formation, course, relations and branches of the nerve involved.

Q 2. A 38-year-old male patient presented to the emergency department after sustaining a sharp knife wound on the medial aspect middle part of the right forearm. On clinical examination, the Froment's test was positive.
   a. Which nerve is involved in this case?
   b. Discuss the formation, course, relations and branches of the nerve involved.
   c. Explain Froment's test and its significance.
   (Hint: Ulnar nerve)

Q 3. A 24-year-old male presented with inability to extend his right wrist for last one day. There was a history of sleeping with right arm hanging on armrest of the chair for a few hours in the night.
   a. Name the nerve compressed in the above-mentioned case.
   b. Mention the course and branches of this nerve.
   (Hint: Radial nerve)

Q 4. Describe the following:
   a. Radial artery in the forearm
   b. Ulnar nerve in hand

Q 5. Write a short note on:
   a. Flexor retinaculum of hand
   b. First carpometacarpal joint
   c. Carpal tunnel syndrome
   d. Superficial palmar arch
   e. Deep palmar arch
   f. Anatomical snuffbox
   g. Lumbricals of hand
   h. Dupuytren's contracture
   i. Whitlow
   j. Midpalmar spaces
   k. Thenar space of hand
   l. Extensor retinaculum of hand

eSmartQuiz

Joints of Upper Limb

CLINICOANATOMICAL PROBLEMS

Clinical Case 1

A 65-year-old woman presents to the emergency department with severe pain and swelling in her right wrist after falling on ground. On clinical examination, there is deformity and tenderness over the right wrist, with noticeable swelling and bruising. The patient is unable to move her wrist and hand without significant pain.

The X-rays reveal a distal radius fracture with dorsal displacement of distal segment, creating a characteristic "dinner fork" deformity.

1. What is the name of this radius bone fracture?
2. In this case, why there is posterior displacement of distal fragment of radius?

Explanation

1. ______________________________

2. ______________________________

Clinical Case 2

A 28-year-old professional boxer presents to the emergency department following a recent boxing match. He had complaints of severe pain and limited range of motion in his right shoulder after receiving a forceful blow to the shoulder during the match. On examination, there is noticeable asymmetry and prominence of the right shoulder compared to the left. The patient is unable to move his right arm without significant pain and apprehension. A physical examination and history suggest a potential shoulder dislocation.

1. Which is the common dislocation of the shoulder?
2. What investigation will you suggest to differentiate fracture of humerus and dislocation of shoulder?
3. Which nerve commonly gets damaged in shoulder dislocation and why?

Explanation

1. ______________________________

2. ______________________________

3. ______________________________

PRACTICE FIGURES

(Label the practice figures)

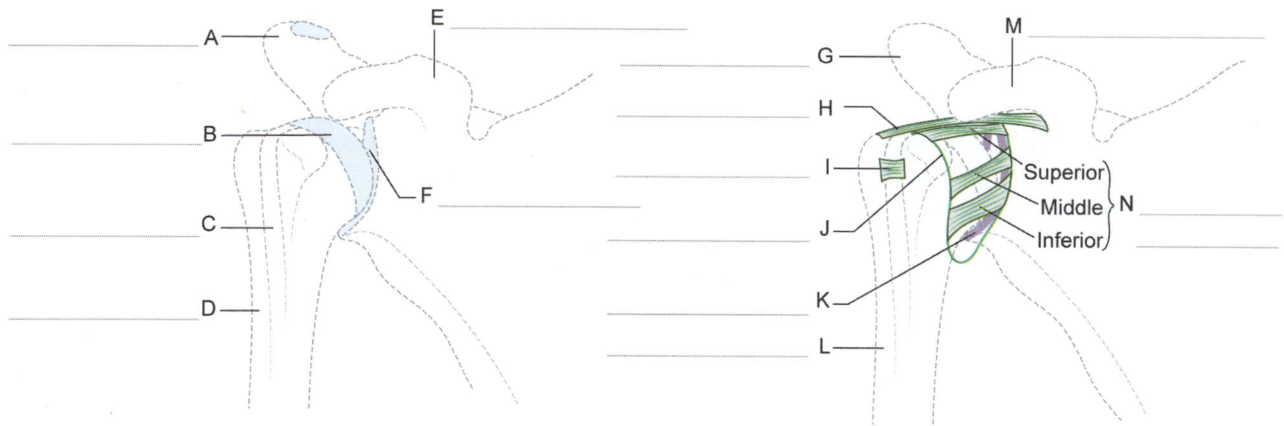

Practice Figure 10.1: Articular surfaces and ligaments of shoulder joint

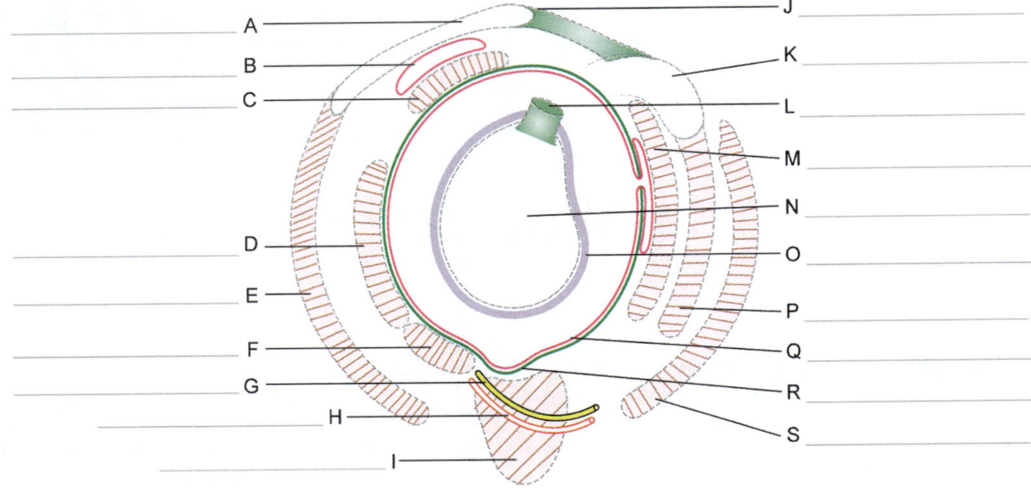

Practice Figure 10.2: Relations of shoulder joint

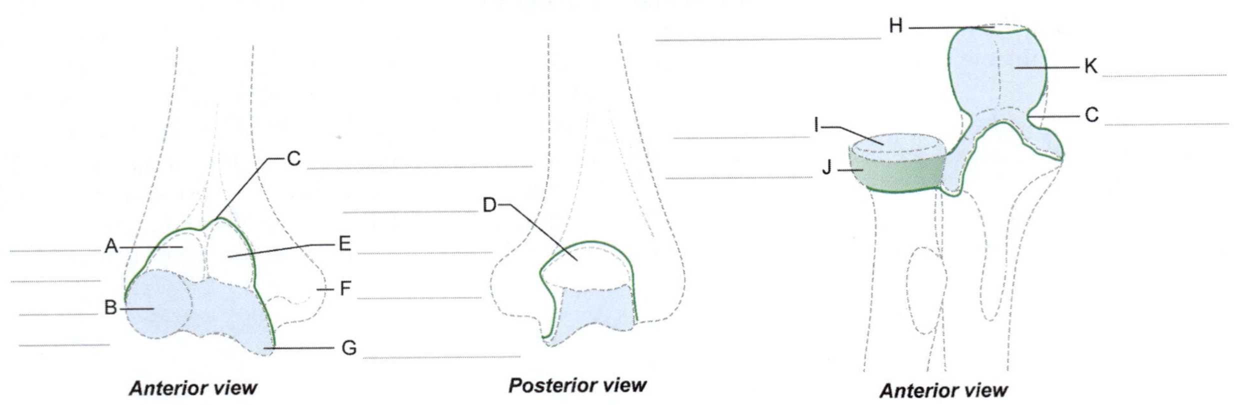

Practice Figure 10.3: Attachment of capsular ligament of elbow joint

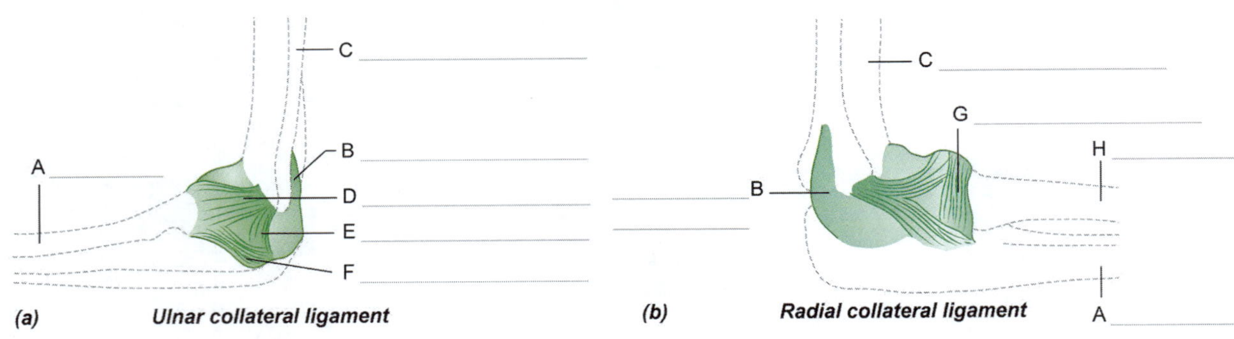

Practice Figure 10.4: Ulnar and radial collateral ligaments

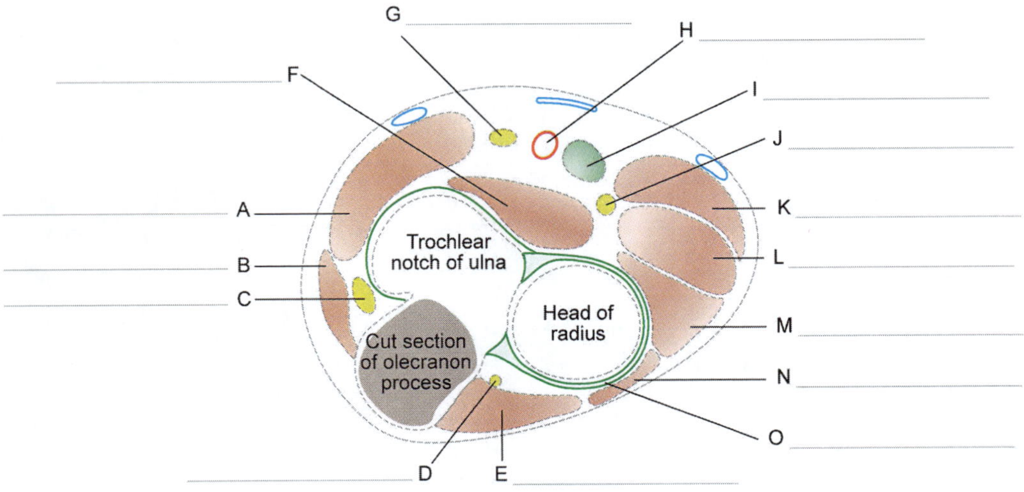

Practice Figure 10.5: Relations of elbow joint (superior view, section passing through the cavity of elbow joint)

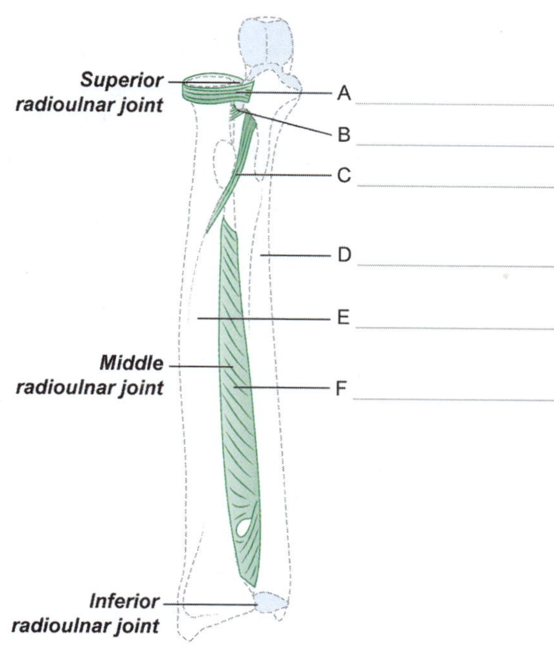

Practice Figure 10.6: Ligaments of radioulnar joints (right, anterior view)

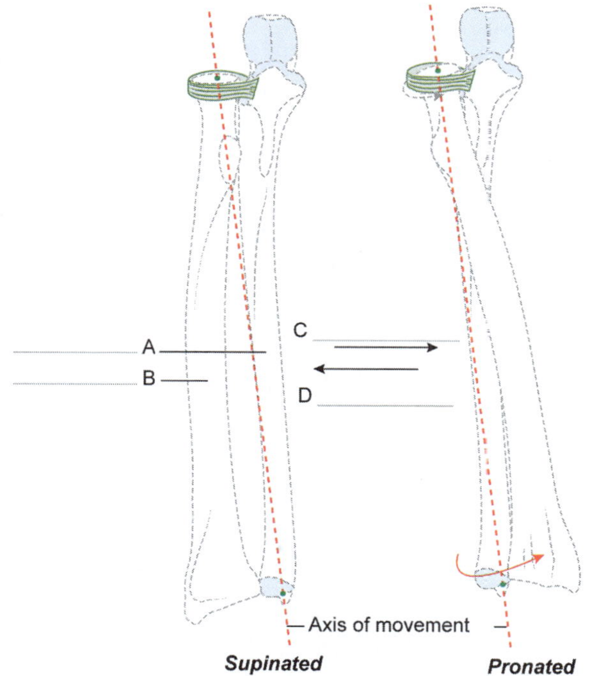

Practice Figure 10.7: Supination and pronation (right)

MULTIPLE CHOICE QUESTIONS

(Tick the single best correct option)

1. Name the clinical condition given below:

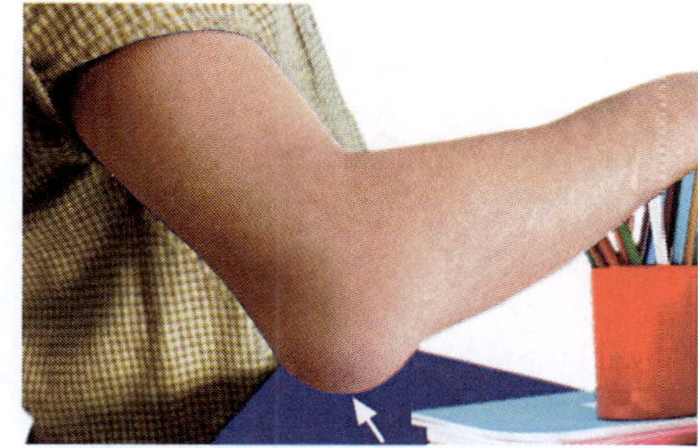

a. Students elbow b. Elbow dislocation
c. Golfer's elbow d. Tennis elbow

2. All of the following muscles produce the abduction at the wrist, EXCEPT:
   a. Flexor carpi radialis
   b. Extensor carpi radialis longus
   c. Extensor carpi radialis brevis
   d. Extensor carpi ulnaris
3. Head of radius is surrounded by ________.
   a. Ulnar collateral ligament
   b. Radial collateral ligament
   c. Quadrate membrane
   d. Annular ligament
4. Tennis elbow occurs due to inflammation of ________ ligament.
   a. Ulnar collateral b. Radial collateral
   c. Quadrate d. Annular
5. Sternoclavicular joint is ________ variety of synovial joint.
   a. Plane b. Saddle
   c. Gliding d. Ellipsoid
6. Acromioclavicular joint is ________ variety of synovial joint.
   a. Plane b. Saddle
   c. Gliding d. Ellipsoid
7. All of the following muscles produce external rotation at the glenohumeral joint, EXCEPT:
   a. Deltoid b. Infraspinatus
   c. Teres minor d. Teres major
8. The skin over the tip of the shoulder is supplied by ________ roots.
   a. C1 and C2 b. C3 and C4
   c. C5 and C6 d. C7 and C8
9. How many metacarpals articulate with the capitate?
   a. Metacarpals 1, 2 b. Metacarpals 2, 3, 4
   c. Metacarpals 1, 2, 3 d. Metacarpals 3, 4, 5
10. First carpometacarpal joint is ________ variety of synovial joint.
    a. Plane b. Saddle
    c. Gliding d. Ellipsoid
11. Medial collateral ligament of elbow joint is closely related to:
    a. Tendon of biceps brachii
    b. Median nerve
    c. Ulnar nerve
    d. Brachial artery
12. Identify the structure marked by X.

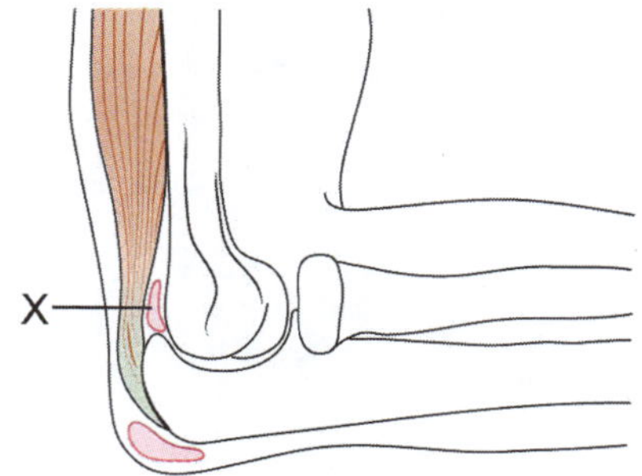

    a. Bicipitoradial bursa
    b. Subcutaneous olecranon bursa
    c. Subtendinous olecranon bursa
    d. Subscapular bursa

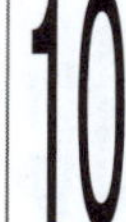

13. Name the actions at the first carpometacarpal joint shown in the following figure.

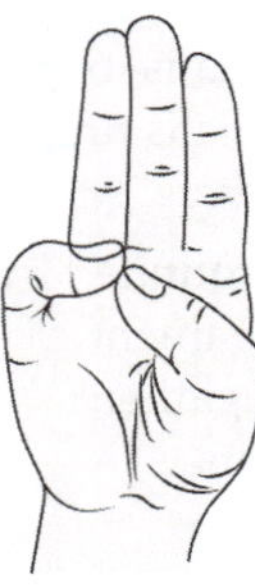

a. Flexion
b. Extension
c. Abduction
d. Opposition

14. All of the following muscles are involved in producing the action at the wrist joint shown in the following figure, EXCEPT:

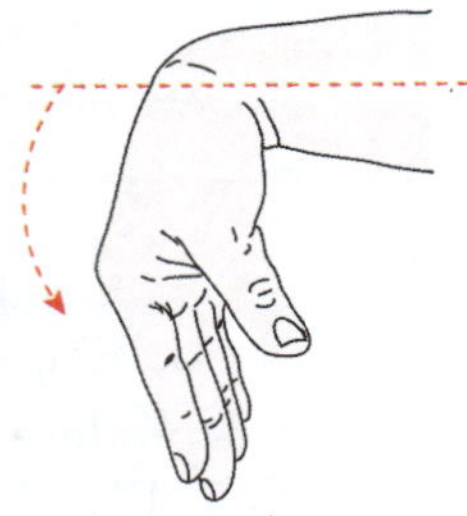

a. Flexor carpi radialis
b. Flexor carpi ulnaris
c. Palmaris longus
d. Brachioradialis

15. Identify the clinical condition shown in the following radiograph.

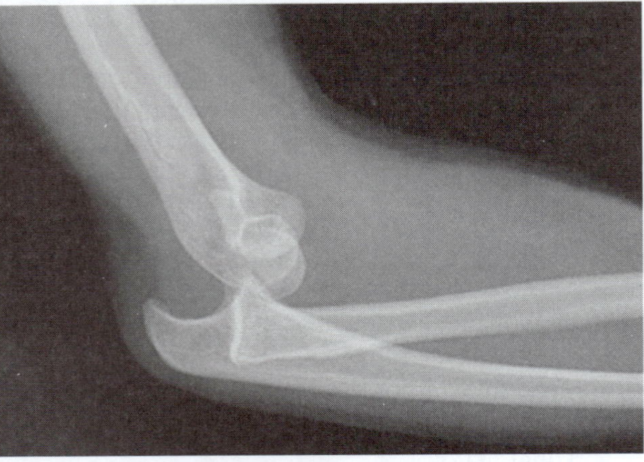

a. Fracture of humerus
b. Dislocation of ulna
c. Subluxation of radius
d. Pulled elbow

QUESTION BANK

(Use separate copy to solve the following questions)

Q 1. Describe the following joints under the following headings: Type and bones forming the joint; Ligaments and relations; Blood supply and nerve supply; Movements and the muscles involved in the movement; and applied aspects
   a. Shoulder joint
   b. Elbow joint
   c. Wrist joint

Q 2. Write a short note on:
   a. Carrying angle
   b. Movements of the thumb with muscles responsible for these movements
   c. First metacarpophalangeal joint
   d. Frozen shoulder
   e. Radioulnar joints
   f. Interosseous membrane of forearm

Q 3. Differences between superior and inferior radioulnar joints.

Surface Marking and Radiological Anatomy of Upper Limb

eSmartQuiz

PRACTICE FIGURES

(Label the practice figures)

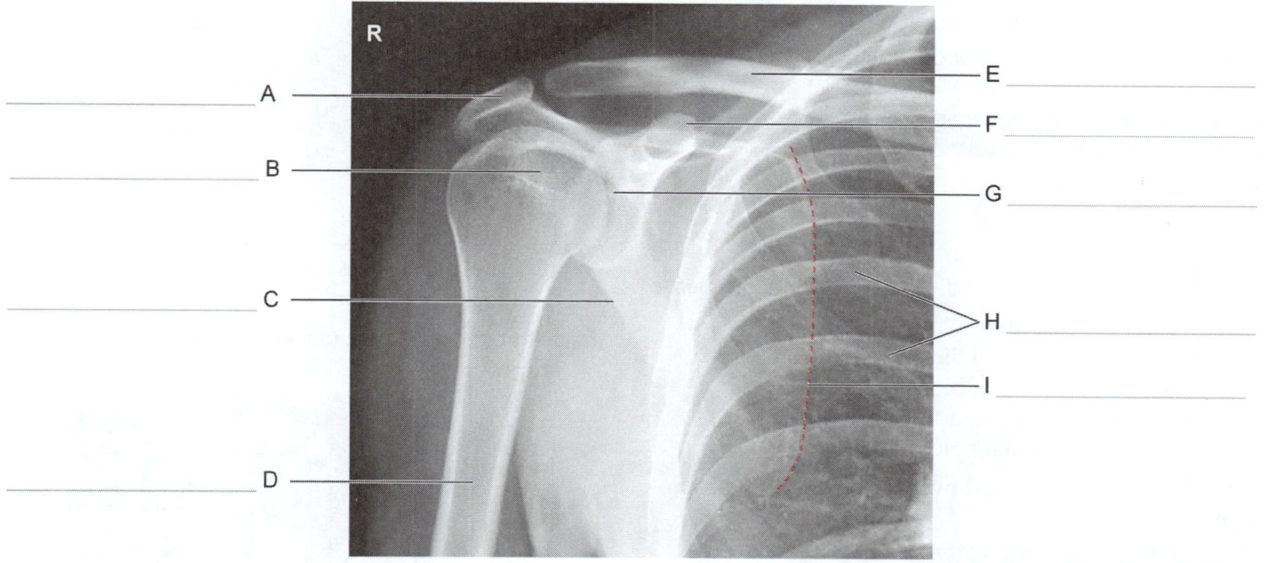

Practice Figure 11.1: Anteroposterior view of the shoulder joint

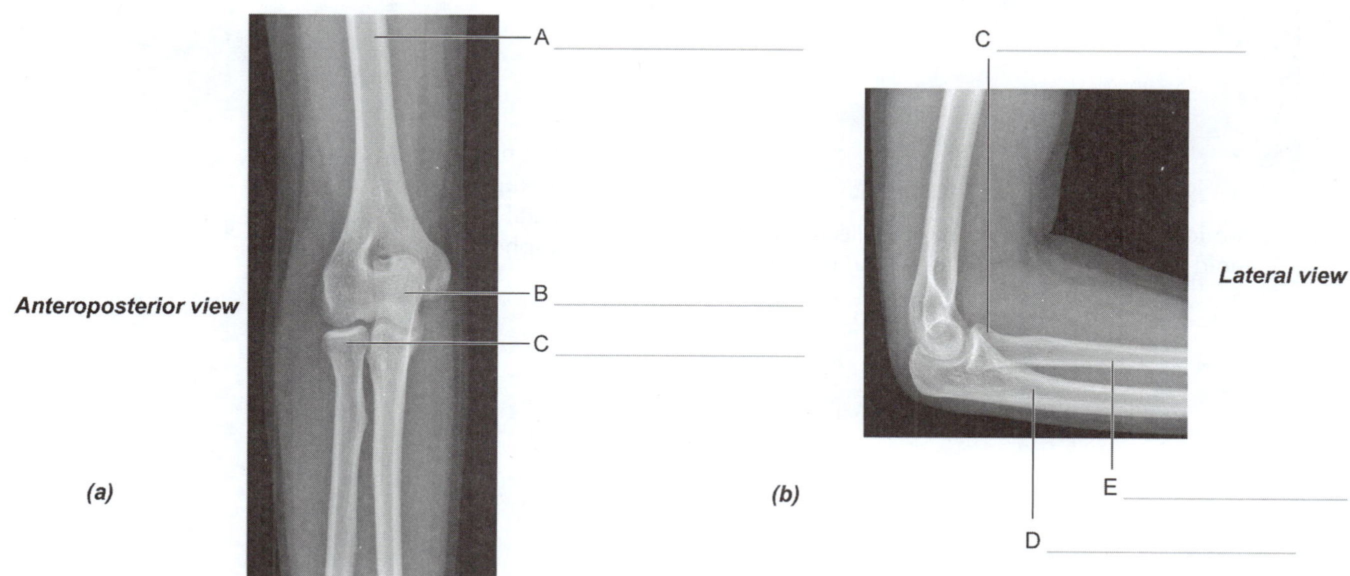

Practice Figure 11.2a and b: Radiograph of elbow joint

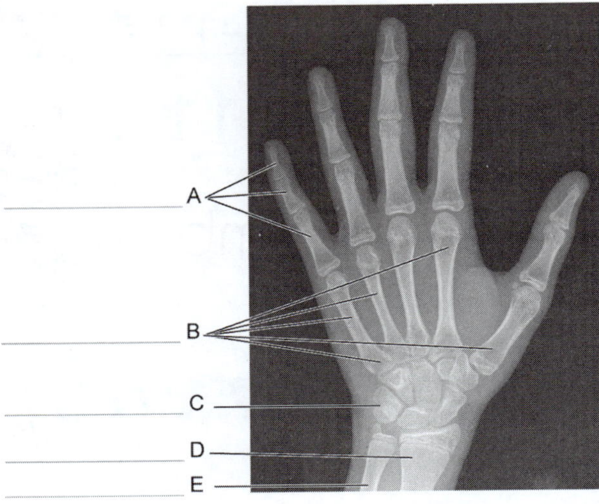

Practice Figure 11.3: Anteroposterior view of hand

MULTIPLE CHOICE QUESTIONS

(Tick the single best correct option)

1. Brachial artery is crossed by ____________.
   a. Median nerve b. Ulnar nerve
   c. Radial nerve d. Musculocutaneous nerve
2. Brachial artery is palpated ____________.
   a. Medial to the tendon of biceps brachii
   b. Lateral to the tendon of biceps brachii
   c. Behind the medial epicondyle
   d. Anterior to the medial epicondyle
3. Name the structure marked by X in the following radiograph.

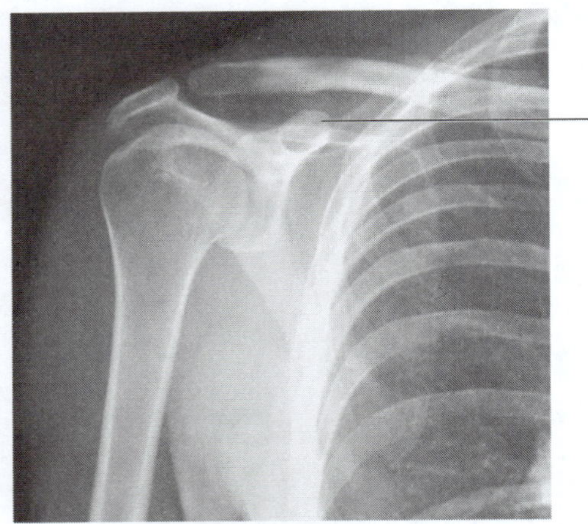

   a. Acromion b. Tip of coracoid process
   c. Glenoid cavity d. Lateral end of clavicle
4. Name the structure marked by X in the following radiograph.

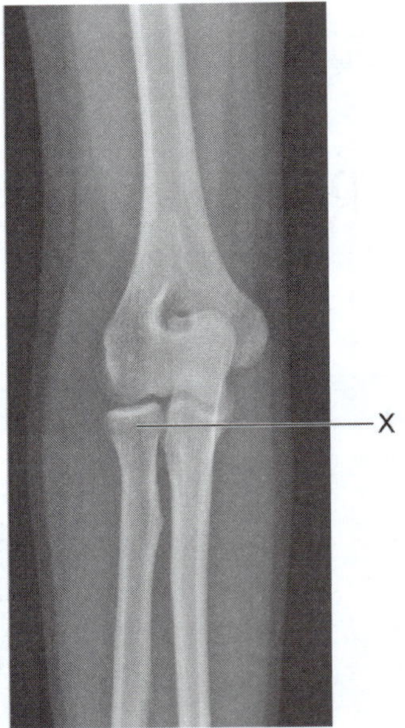

   a. Head of radius
   b. Olecranon process
   c. Coronoid process
   d. Trochlea
5. Name the structure marked by X in the following radiograph.

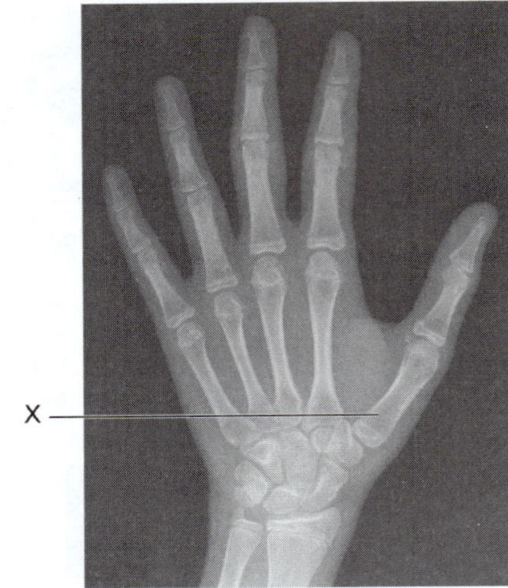

   a. First metacarpal
   b. Proximal phalanx of thumb
   c. Distal phalanx of thumb
   d. Scaphoid

Thorax

Chapter

12

eSmartQuiz

Introduction

CLINICOANATOMICAL PROBLEMS

Clinical Case 1

A 55-year-old man presents to the clinic with a complaints of persistent hiccups for the past two days. He describes the hiccups as occurring every few minutes. He had history of heartburn, often after eating or when lying down. Clinical examination revealed regular, rhythmic contractions of the diaphragm, consistent with hiccups. A complete blood count and biochemical tests were within normal limits. The clinician diagnosed this case as gastroesophageal reflux disease (GERD).

1. What is the cause of hiccups in this case?
2. What nerve is responsible for these hiccups?
3. Enlist any one another cause of hiccups.

Explanation

1. ______________________

2. ______________________

3. ______________________

Clinical Case 2

A newborn infant is brought to the paediatric clinic for the signs of respiratory distress shortly after birth. On physical examination, there are signs of respiratory distress, including tachypnoea (rapid breathing), retractions (visible sinking of the chest wall during breathing) and cyanosis (bluish discolouration of the skin). Auscultation of the chest revealed decreased breath sounds on the left side. The paediatrician suspected a congenital diaphragmatic hernia (CDH). Chest X-rays are obtained, which confirm the diagnosis of a posterolateral diaphragmatic hernia. The X-rays revealed liver, spleen and coils of intestine in the chest cavity, with displacement of the mediastinum to the contralateral side.

1. What is the name of this hernia?
2. Is it common on right or left?
3. Which is the commonest congenital diaphragmatic hernia?

1. ______________________

2. ______________________

3. ______________________

PRACTICE FIGURES

(Label the practice figures)

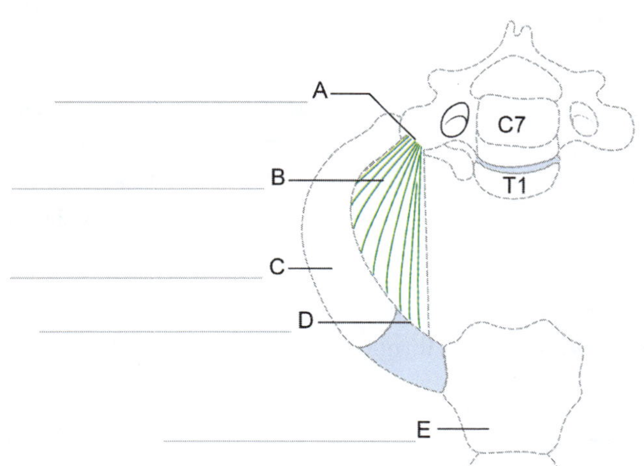

Practice Figure 12.1: The suprapleural membrane

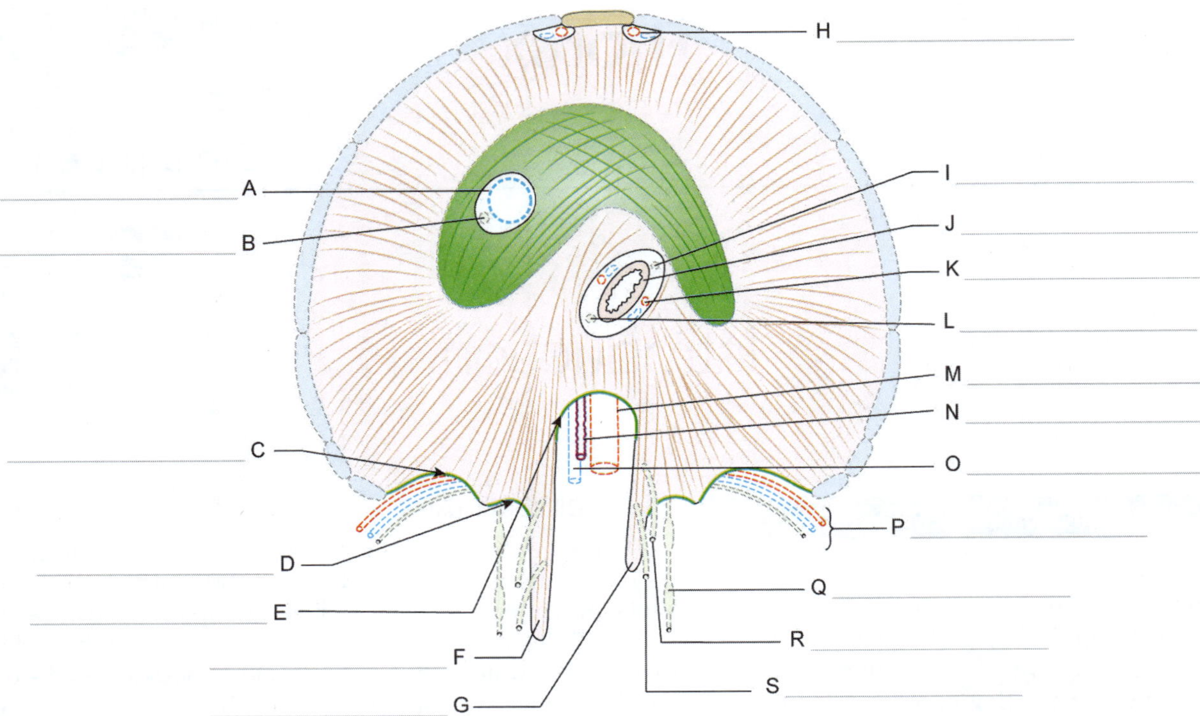

Practice Figure 12.2: Openings in the diaphragm and structures passing through these openings

MULTIPLE CHOICE QUESTIONS

(Tick the single best correct option)

1. The aortic orifice in the diaphragm lies at the ________ level of vertebra.
   a. T6 b. T8
   c. T10 d. T12
2. All of the following structures enter the neck through thoracic inlet, EXCEPT:
   a. Left common carotid artery
   b. Left subclavian artery
   c. Trachea
   d. Descending aorta
3. Suprapleural membrane is attached to ________.
   a. Anterior aspect of clavicle
   b. Upper border of scapula
   c. Inner margin of 1st rib
   d. Transverse process of 6th cervical vertebra
4. Which of the following structures is related superiorly to the suprapleural membrane?
   a. Subclavian vessels
   b. Trachea
   c. Cervical pleura
   d. Apex of the lung
5. The cervical rib may compress the ________ of brachial plexus.
   a. Lower trunk b. Upper trunk
   c. Lateral cord d. Medial cord
6. Which of the following structures does not pass through the aortic orifice of the diaphragm?
   a. Aorta b. Thoracic duct
   c. Sympathetic trunk d. Azygos vein
7. Which of the following structures pass through the oesophageal orifice of the diaphragm?
   a. Right vagus nerve
   b. Right phrenic nerve
   c. Sympathetic trunk
   d. Lesser splanchnic nerves
8. ________ is affected in thoracic inlet syndrome.
   a. C7 b. C8
   c. T1 d. T2
9. Which structure passes deep to the lateral arcuate ligament?
   a. Superior epigastric artery
   b. Subcostal vessels
   c. Greater splanchnic nerves
   d. Left phrenic nerve
10. Which structure passes through the space of Larrey?
    a. Superior epigastric artery
    b. Sympathetic trunk
    c. Greater splanchnic nerves
    d. Left phrenic nerve

QUESTION BANK

(Use separate copy to solve the following questions)

Q 1. Enumerate the landmarks at the level of sternal angle.

Q 2. Enumerate various structures passing through the inlet of thorax.

Q 3. Write short notes on:
   a. Cervical rib
   b. Main openings in the thoracoabdominal diaphragm, including their levels and contents
   c. Diaphragmatic hernia

eSmartQuiz

Bones and Joints of Thorax

CLINICOANATOMICAL PROBLEM

Clinical Case 1

A 35-year-old woman presented to the clinic with complaints of numbness, tingling and weakness in her right arm, particularly in the hand and fingers. She reports experiencing these symptoms intermittently for several months, with episodes of worsening during certain activities such as lifting objects or reaching overhead. Additionally, the patient mentions occasional episodes of coldness and discolouration of her right hand. On physical examination, there is evidence of muscle wasting in the right hand (Finding a) and diminished pulses in the right upper extremity (Finding b). The physician suspects thoracic outlet syndrome (TOS) due to cervical rib.

1. What may be the reason for thoracic outlet syndrome?
2. How the cervical rib can be detected?
3. What are the reasons for Findings a and b?

Explanation

1. ______________________________

2. ______________________________

3. Finding a: ______________________________

Finding b: ______________________________

PRACTICE FIGURES

(Label the practice figures)

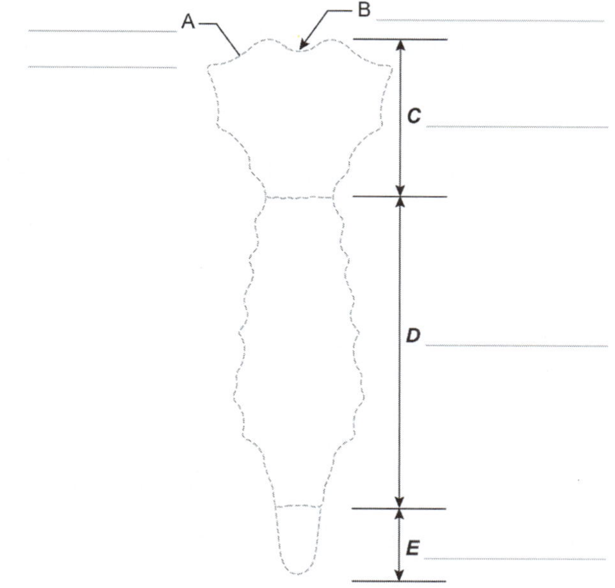

Practice Figure 13.1: The sternum: Anterior aspect

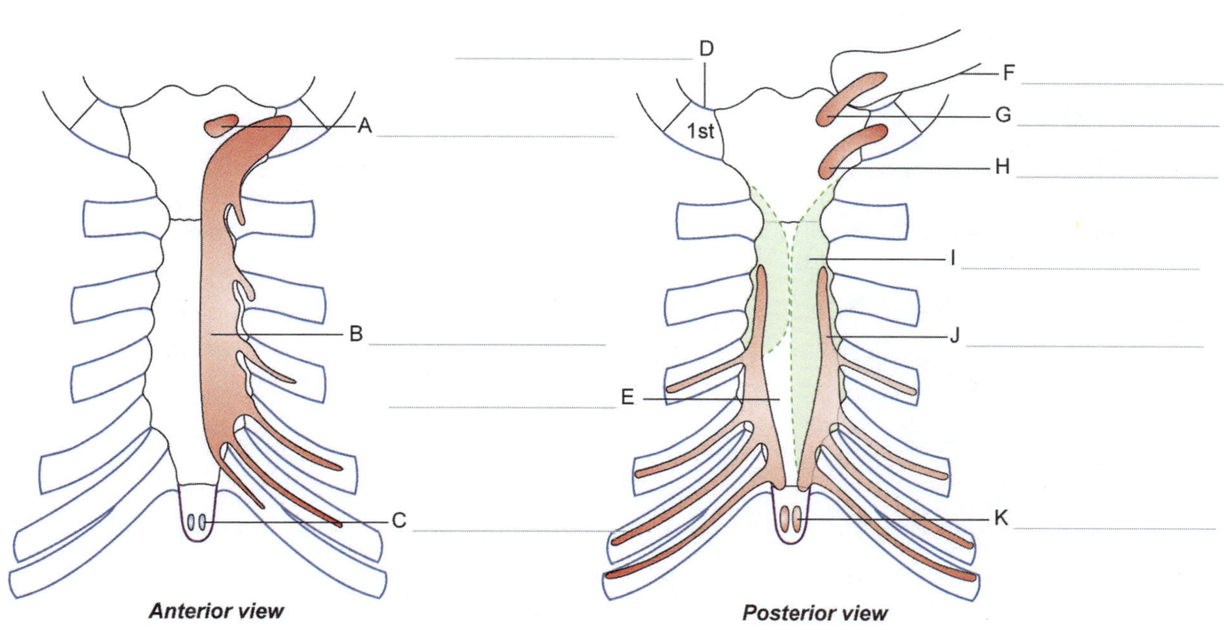

Practice Figure 13.2: Attachments of sternum

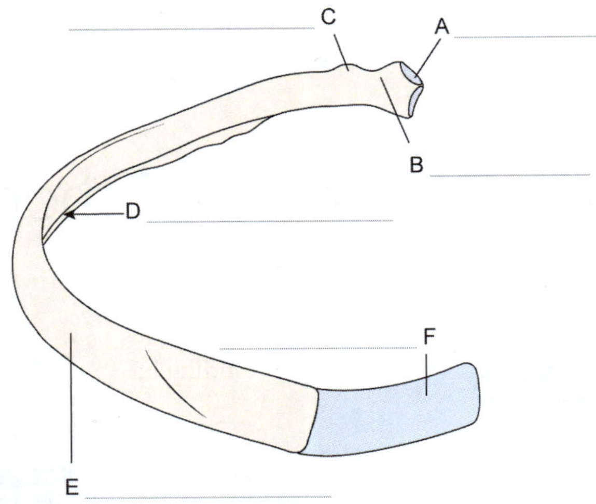

Practice Figure 13.3: Typical rib (right)

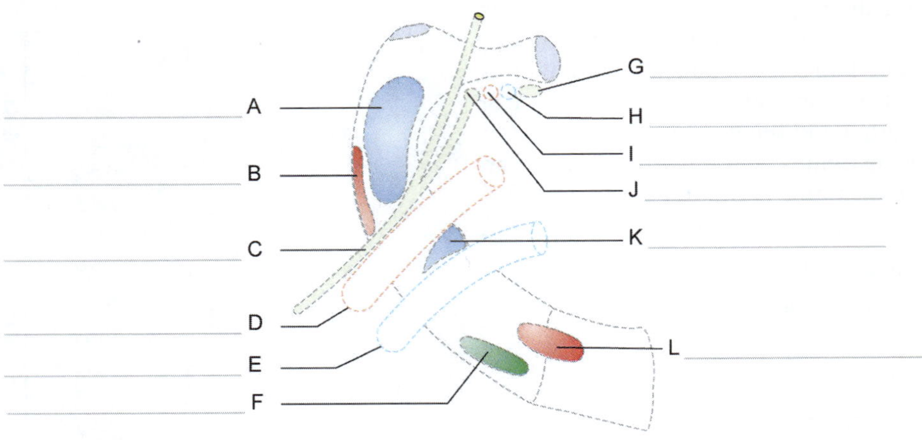

Practice Figure 13.4: Superior view of the first rib

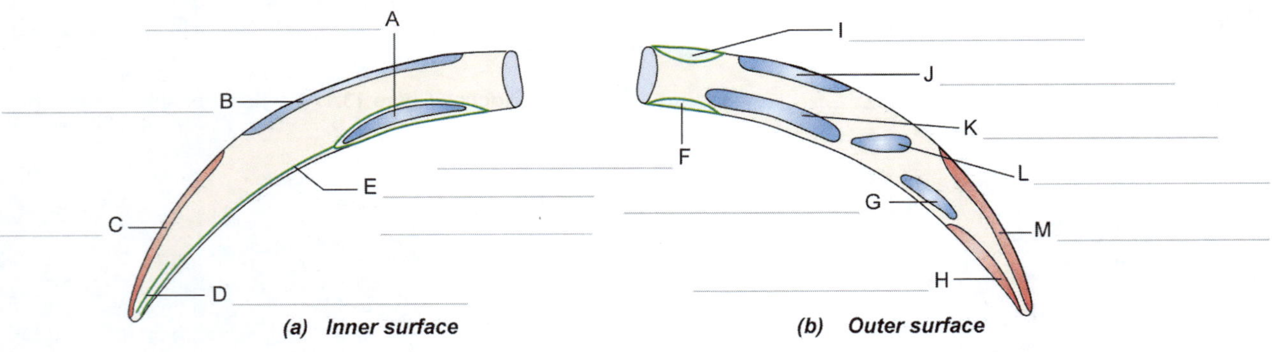

Practice Figure 13.5: Twelfth rib: (a) Inner surface (anterior aspect) and (b) outer surface (posterior aspect)

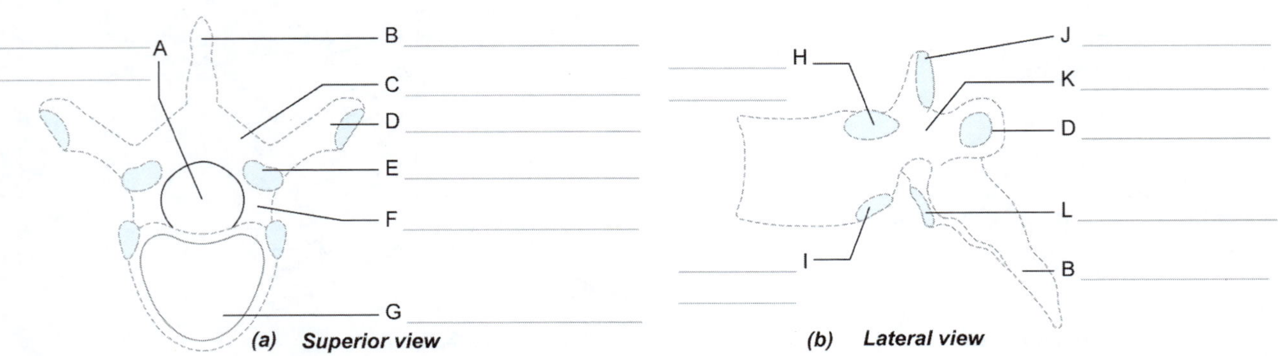

Practice Figure 13.6: Typical thoracic vertebra: (a) Superior view and (b) lateral view

Superior complete costal facet
T1
Spinous process
Superior costal demifacet
T9
Single, complete costal facet
T10
Single, complete costal facet
T11
Transverse process with three tubercles
T12

T1 ______________________

T9 ______________________

T10 ______________________

T11 ______________________

T12 ______________________

Practice Figure 13.7: Features of atypical thoracic vertebrae

MULTIPLE CHOICE QUESTIONS

(Tick the single best correct option)

1. All of the following structures are related to the neck of the 1st rib anteriorly, EXCEPT
   a. Sympathetic trunk
   b. Superior intercostal vein
   c. Superior intercostal artery
   d. Ventral ramus of first thoracic nerve
2. The first chondrosternal joint is a ____________ joint.
   a. Plane synovial joint
   b. Primary cartilaginous joint
   c. Secondary cartilaginous joint
   d. Fibrous joint
3. ________ muscle holds down the 12th rib during respiration.
   a. Transverse abdominus b. External oblique
   c. Internal oblique d. Quadratus lumborum
4. Which of the following ribs articulates with one vertebra only?
   a. First b. Second
   c. Third d. Fourth
5. The most characteristic feature of the thoracic vertebrae is:
   a. The body is heart-shaped
   b. The spine is oblique
   c. The body has costal facets
   d. Vertebral foramen is small and circular
6. The lower larger facet on the head of a typical rib articulates with the demifacet on:
   a. Inferior part of corresponding vertebrae
   b. Superior part of corresponding vertebrae
   c. Inferior part of vertebra above the corresponding vertebrae
   d. Superior part of vertebra below the corresponding vertebrae
7. Which of the following is the vertebrochondral rib?
   a. First b. Tenth
   c. Eleventh d. Twelfth
8. Which of the following ribs has two facets at the head?
   a. First rib b. Second rib
   c. Eleventh rib d. Twelfth rib
9. All of the following are true about the twelfth rib, EXCEPT:
   a. Head has single facet
   b. Anterior end is free and pointed
   c. Neck, angle and costal groove are absent
   d. Tubercle has articular facet
10. Identify the vertebra shown in the following figure.

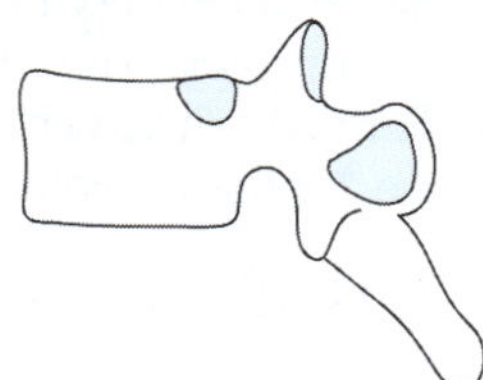

   a. T9 b. T10
   c. T11 d. T12
11. Identify the ligament marked by X.

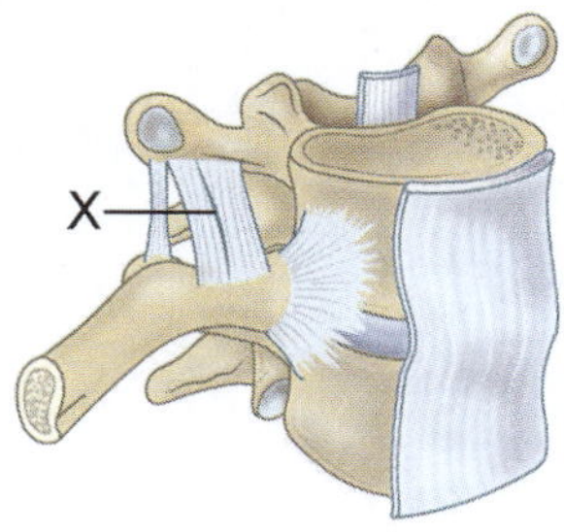

   a. Lateral costotransverse b. Inferior costotransverse
   c. Superior costotransverse d. Intertransverse

QUESTION BANK

(Use separate copy to solve the following questions)

Q 1. In Pranayama, to increase the lung capacity, what are the movements and the diameters increased during the respiration.

Q 2. Draw the diagram of first rib showing its relations.

Q 3. What are the changes occurring at the sternal angle?

Q 4. List the typical and atypical ribs and vertebrae.

Q 5. List the identification features of typical thoracic vertebrae.

Q 6. Write a short note on intervertebral disc.

Chapter

14

eSmartQuiz

Walls of Thorax

CLINICOANATOMICAL PROBLEMS

Clinical Case 1

A 55-year-old male construction worker came to the OPD with complaints of progressively worsening back pain over the past six months. He described the pain as dull and constant, aggravated by movement and relieved partially by rest. He also reported that over the previous two months, he had been occasionally having low-grade fevers and night sweats. On clinical examination, there was tenderness and stiffness in the thoracic spine region, particularly around the T6–T8 vertebrae, along with a restricted range of motion. Neurological examination reveals no focal deficits.

X-ray of the thoracic spines showed loss of vertebral height and destruction of the T6–T8 vertebral bodies with perispinal soft tissue shadow.

Blood tests suggested elevated ESR (erythrocyte sedimentation rate) and CRP (C-reactive protein). The physician diagnosed him with tuberculosis of the thoracic vertebrae.

1. What is another name for the tuberculosis of the thoracic vertebrae?
2. What is the reason for the perispinal soft tissue shadow?
3. What is cold abscess?

Explanation

1. ______
2. ______
3. ______

Clinical Case 2

For thoracocentesis, a resident inserted a needle near the lower border of the 8th rib at the right anterior axillary line and withdraws 15 ml of fluid. The next day, during the rounds, the patient complained of tingling and numbness of the skin of his chest from the level of the 8th rib down towards the umbilicus on the right side.

1. What is thoracocentesis?
2. What should be the ideal site of needle insertion in the 8th intercostal space in the midaxillary line?
3. Why the patient complained about tingling and numbness of the skin of his chest from the level of the 8th rib down towards the umbilicus on the right side?

Explanation

1. ______

2. ______

3. ______

PRACTICE FIGURES

(Label the practice figures)

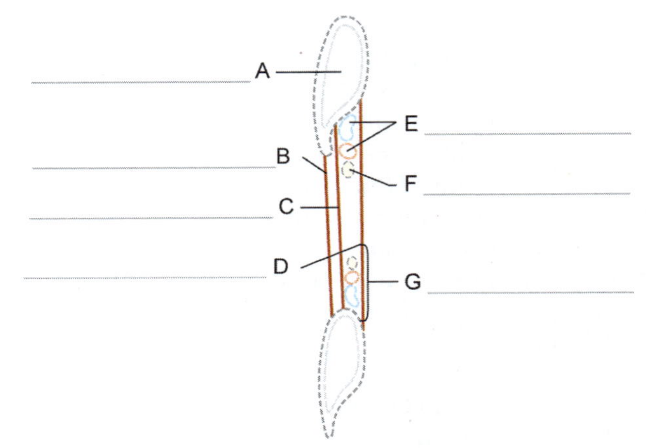

Practice Figure 14.1: Section of typical intercostal space with neurovascular bundle and its collateral branches

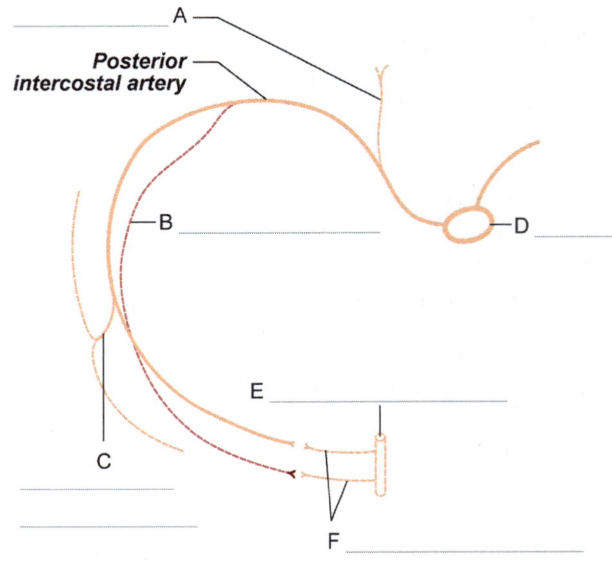

Practice Figure 14.2: Scheme showing the intercostal arteries

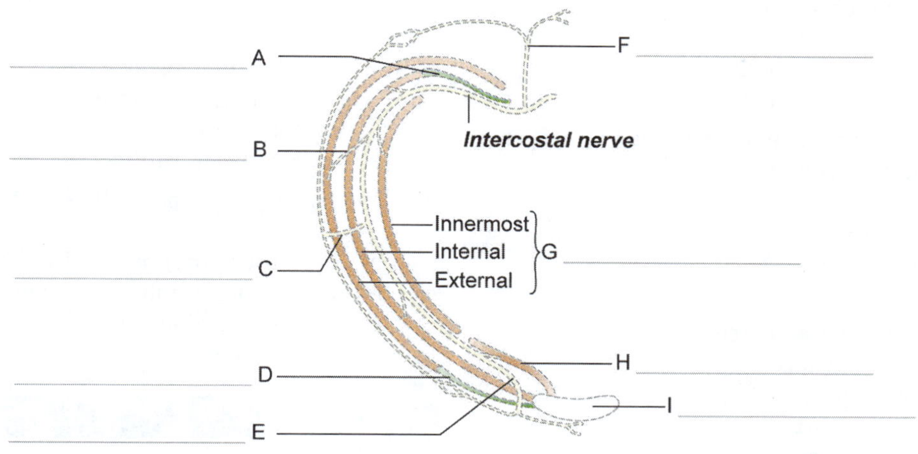

Practice Figure 14.3: Course and branches of typical intercostal nerve (right)

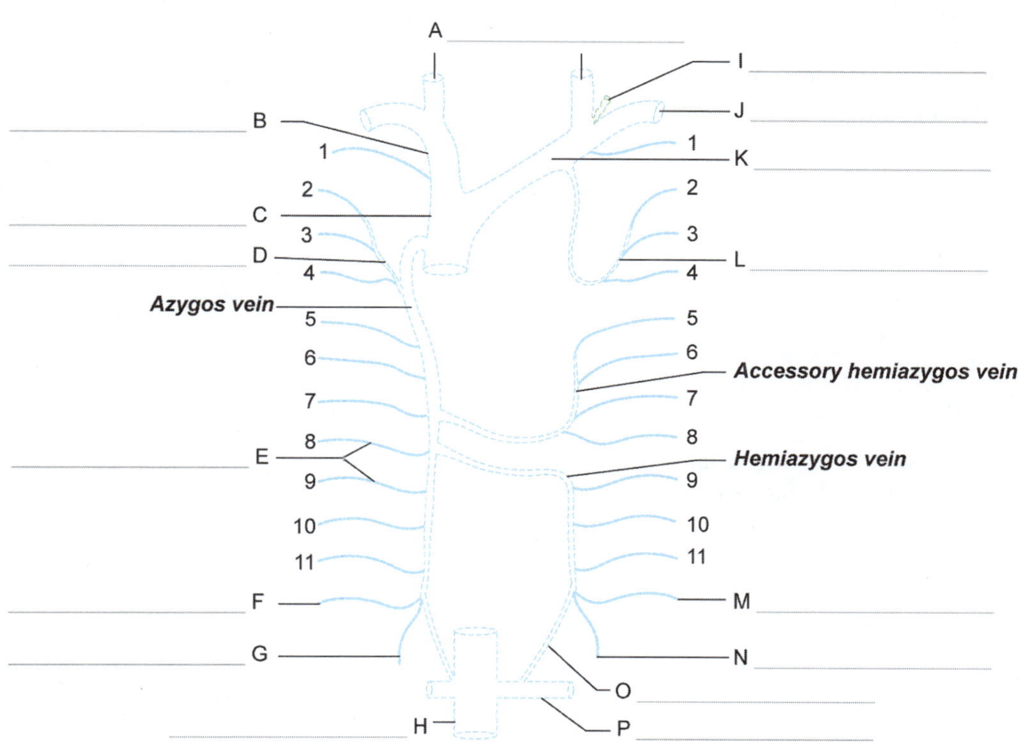

Practice Figure 14.4: Drainage of posterior intercostal veins

MULTIPLE CHOICE QUESTIONS

(Tick the single best correct option)

1. Anterior intercostal membrane is the continuation of ____________ muscle.
   a. External intercostal muscle
   b. Internal intercostal muscle
   c. Intercostalis intimi muscle
   d. Subcostalis muscle
2. Which of the following muscles is attached to the floor of the costal groove?
   a. External intercostal muscle
   b. Internal intercostal muscle
   c. Intercostalis intimi muscle
   d. Subcostalis muscle
3. All of the following are atypical intercostal nerves, *Except*:
   a. 1st b. 2nd
   c. 6th d. 7th
4. Identify the structure marked X in the following figure.

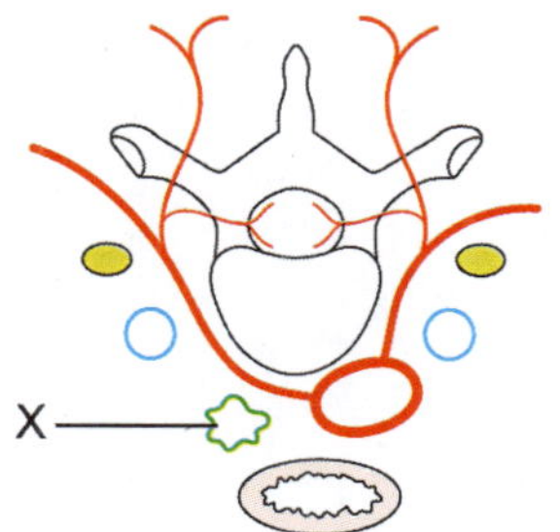

   a. Azygos vein b. Hemiazygos vein
   c. Thoracic duct d. Posterior intercostal artery

5. Which posterior intercostal veins of left side drain into accessory hemiazygos vein?
   a. 1st to 4th
   b. 2nd to 4th
   c. 5th to 8th
   d. 9th to 11th
6. Which of the following movements of the thoracic cage may occur during respiration?
   a. Pump handle movement
   b. Bucket handle movement
   c. Piston movement
   d. All of the above
7. Musculophrenic artery is a branch of:
   a. Superior epigastric artery
   b. Internal thoracic artery
   c. Superior thoracic artery
   d. Anterior intercostal artery
8. Which of the following muscles is required for expiration during quite breathing?
   a. Diaphragm
   b. External intercostal
   c. Scalene muscles
   d. None of the above-mentioned muscles are required.
9. Identify the following muscle marked with X.

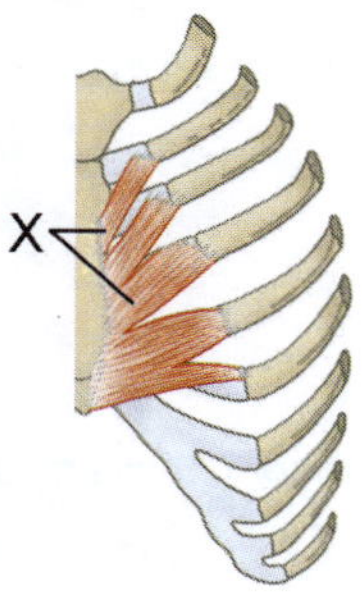

   a. Intercostalis intimus
   b. Subcostalis
   c. Levatores costarum
   d. Sternocostalis
10. The first posterior intercostal artery is the branch of the ____________.
   a. Superior intercostal artery
   b. Descending thoracic aorta
   c. Internal thoracic artery
   d. Costocervical trunk
11. The first right posterior intercostal vein opens into the ____________.
   a. Right brachiocephalic vein
   b. Right superior intercostal vein
   c. Right subclavian vein
   d. Azygos vein

QUESTION BANK

(Use separate copy to solve the following questions)

Q 1. Actions of intercostal muscles
Q 2. Typical intercostal nerve
Q 3. Typical posterior intercostal artery
Q 4. Azygos vein
Q 5. Thoracocentesis
Q 6. Thoracic sympathetic chain.

Chapter

15

eSmartQuiz

Thoracic Cavity and Pleurae

CLINICOANATOMICAL PROBLEMS

Clinical Case 1

A 62-year-old female presents with worsening shortness of breath, dry cough and sharp right-sided chest pain, accompanied by fatigue and decreased appetite. Clinical examination reveals dyspnoea, tachypnoea and tachycardia. Diminished breath sounds and dullness to percussion are noted over the right lower lung fields, with decreased chest expansion on the right. Chest X-ray shows a large right-sided pleural effusion, obliterating the right costodiaphragmatic recess, causing mediastinal shift to the left and compression of the right lung.

1. What is pleural effusion?
2. What is costodiaphragmatic recess?
3. Normally how the costodiaphragmatic recess appears on X-ray?
4. Name the procedure required to collect the plural fluid for diagnosis.

Explanation

1. ______

2. ______

3. ______

4. ______

Clinical Case 2

A 30-year-old male soldier was brought to the emergency department after sustaining a single gunshot wound to the left side of his chest. Upon arrival, he was conscious but in severe respiratory distress. He complained of sharp chest pain on the left side and difficulty breathing. On clinical examination, he had tachycardia, tachypnoea and hypotension. Auscultation of the chest revealed absent breath sounds on the left side and hyperresonance to percussion. Tracheal deviation away from the affected side was noted. The chest X-ray showed complete collapse of the left lung with mediastinal shift to the right, consistent with tension pneumothorax.

1. What is tension pneumothorax?
2. In this case, why the gunshot injury resulted in the tension pneumothorax?
3. Why there is mediastinal shift to the opposite side?
4. How to relieve the tension pneumothorax?

Explanation

1. ______

2. ______

3. ______

4. ______

PRACTICE FIGURE

(Label the practice figure)

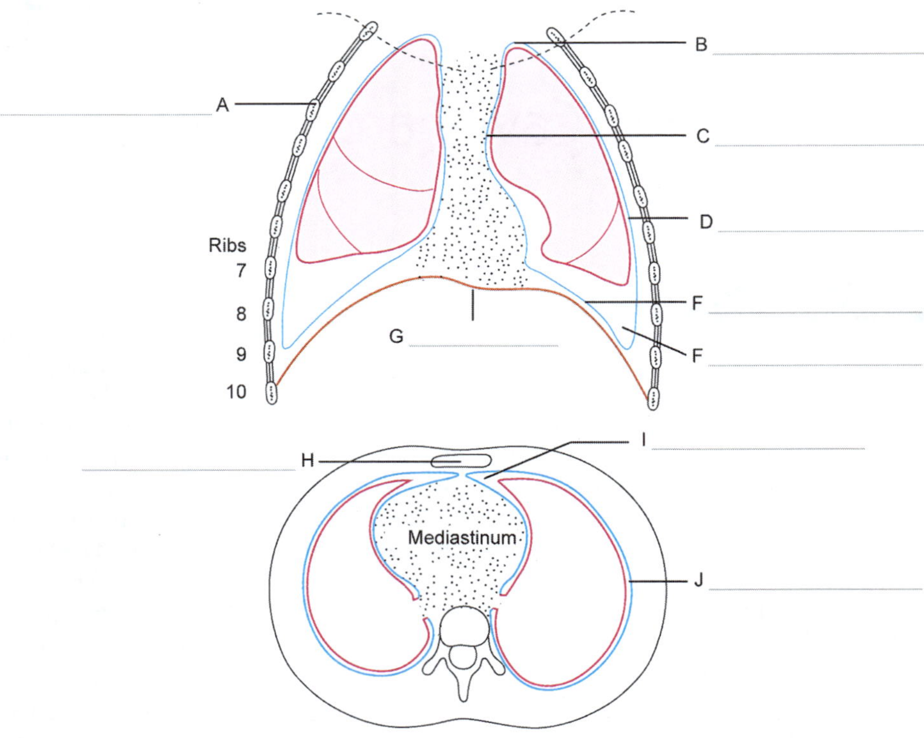

Practice Figure 15.1: Costodiaphragmatic and costomediastinal recesses

MULTIPLE CHOICE QUESTIONS

(Tick the single best correct option)

1. All of the following are true about the parietal pleura, *Except*:
   a. It develops from somatopleuric mesoderm
   b. It is supplied by phrenic nerve
   c. It is supplied by bronchial vessels
   d. It is sensitive to pain and touch
2. Mediastinal pleura is innervated by __________ nerve.
   a. Phrenic b. Intercostal
   c. Vagus d. Subcostal
3. In the midaxillary line the inferior margin of parietal pleura crosses __________ rib.
   a. 6th b. 8th
   c. 10th d. 12th
4. Pleura extends beyond the thoracic cage in the following areas, EXCEPT:
   a. Right xiphicostal angle
   b. Right and left costovertebral angles
   c. Right and left sides of root of neck as cervical dome of pleura
   d. Right and left costodiaphragmatic angles
5. Which of the following is NOT the content of the pulmonary ligament?
   a. Loose areolar tissue
   b. Lymphatics
   c. Accessory bronchial artery
   d. Pulmonary vein
6. All of the following are true about the plural cavity, EXCEPT:
   a. Costodiaphragmatic recess forms most dependent part of the pleural cavity.
   b. Costomediastinal recess lies between costal and mediastinal pleurae.
   c. Left costomediastinal recess is smaller than the right costomediastinal recess.
   d. Costodiaphragmatic recess extends from 10th to 12th ribs in paravertebral line.
7. Normally the intrapleural pressure is ________ mm of Hg.
   a. –4 b. 4
   c. 12 d. –12
8. Empyema is the accumulation of _______ in the plural cavity.
   a. Blood b. Serous fluid
   c. Pus d. Air
9. Name the procedure shown in the following figure.

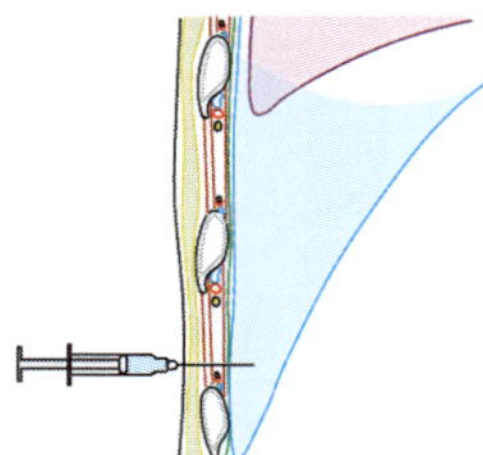

   a. Thoracocentesis b. Pericardiocentesis
   c. Amniocentesis d. Paracentesis
10. The pain from the mediastinal pleura is referred to the shoulder due to __________ segment of spinal cord.
   a. C2 b. C4
   c. C6 d. C8

QUESTION BANK

(Use separate copy to solve the following questions)

Q 1. List the differences between visceral and parietal pleurae.
Q 2. Pleural recesses.
Q 3. Pleural effusion and its anatomical basis.

eSmartQuiz

Lungs

CLINICOANATOMICAL PROBLEMS

Clinical Case 1

A 3-year-old boy was brought to the emergency department due to sudden onset of coughing, choking and respiratory distress. The boy was playing with coins before the beginning of the symptoms. Auscultation of the chest revealed decreased air entry on the right side (Finding a), with wheezing and crackles heard predominantly over the right lung fields. The chest X-ray showed a round, radiopaque foreign body in the right main bronchus, consistent with a coin.

1. What is the anatomical basis for the involvement of the right principal bronchus?
2. What was the cause for the Finding a?
3. What are the potential complications that may occur in this condition?

Explanation

1. ______________________________

2. ______________________________

3. ______________________________

Clinical Case 2

A 60-year-old male patient came to OPD with complaints of severe cough, significant weight loss over the past few months and hoarseness of voice. He has been a chronic smoker for the last 20 years. He reports a persistent cough that is productive of sputum, occasionally tinged with blood. He has noticed a gradual loss of appetite and energy, accompanied by unintentional weight loss. Clinical examination of the chest revealed diminished breath sounds over the left upper lung zone. The chest X-ray showed a mass lesion in the left upper lobe of the lung and mediastinal lymphadenopathy. A biopsy of the lung lesion confirms the diagnosis of bronchogenic adenocarcinoma.

1. Which is the most common factor causing this cancer?
2. Where did the cancer cells metastasis in this case?
3. What is the anatomical basis for the hoarseness of voice?

Explanation

1. ______________________________

2. ______________________________

3. ______________________________

PRACTICE FIGURES

(Label the practice figures)

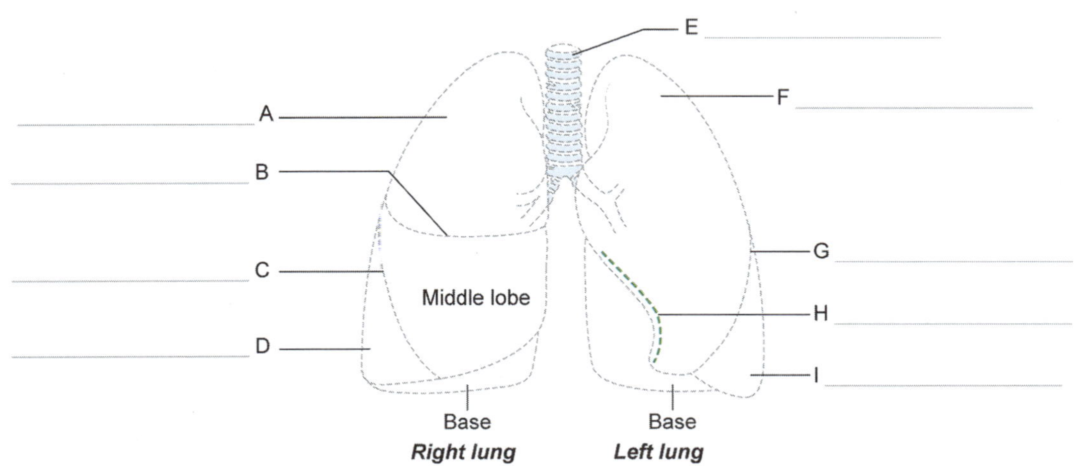

Practice Figure 16.1: The trachea and lungs as seen from the front

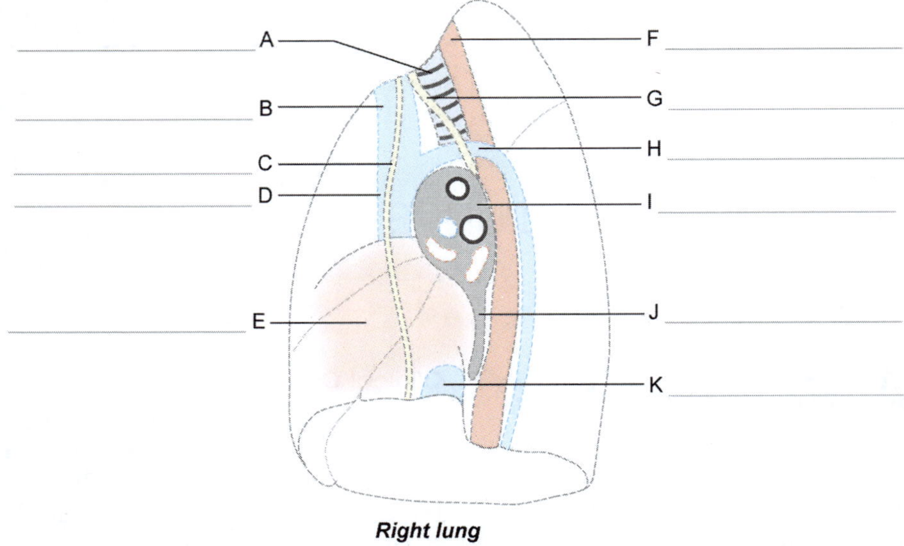

Practice Figure 16.2: Mediastinal surface of right lung

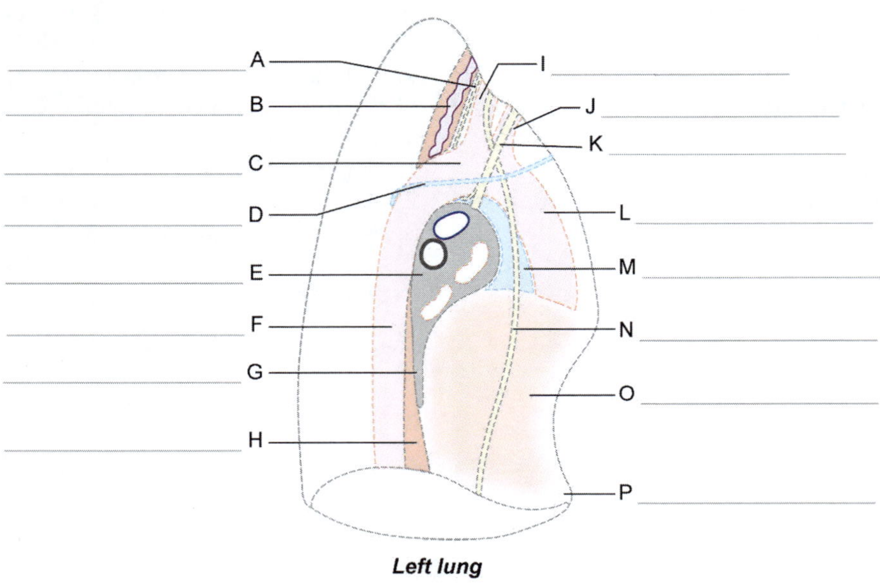

Practice Figure 16.3: Mediastinal surface of left lung

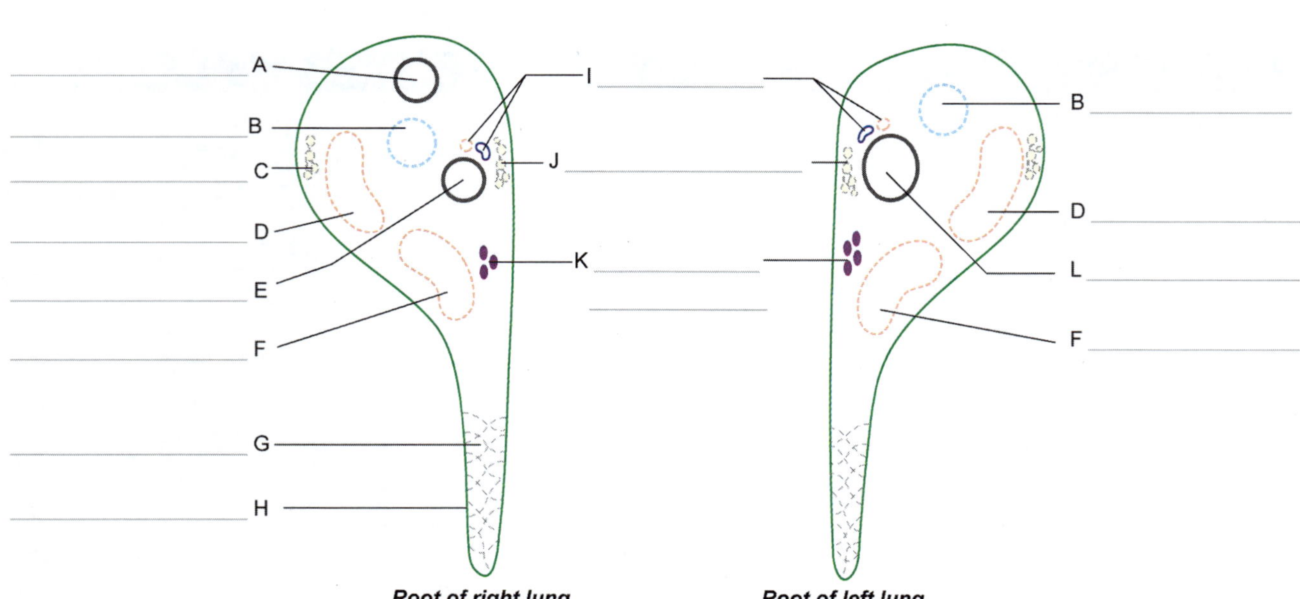

Practice Figure 16.4: Roots of the right and left lungs

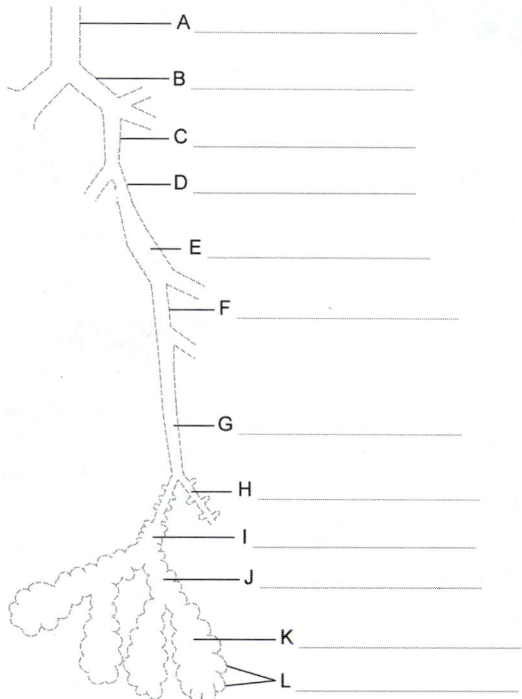

Practice Figure 16.5: Bronchial tree

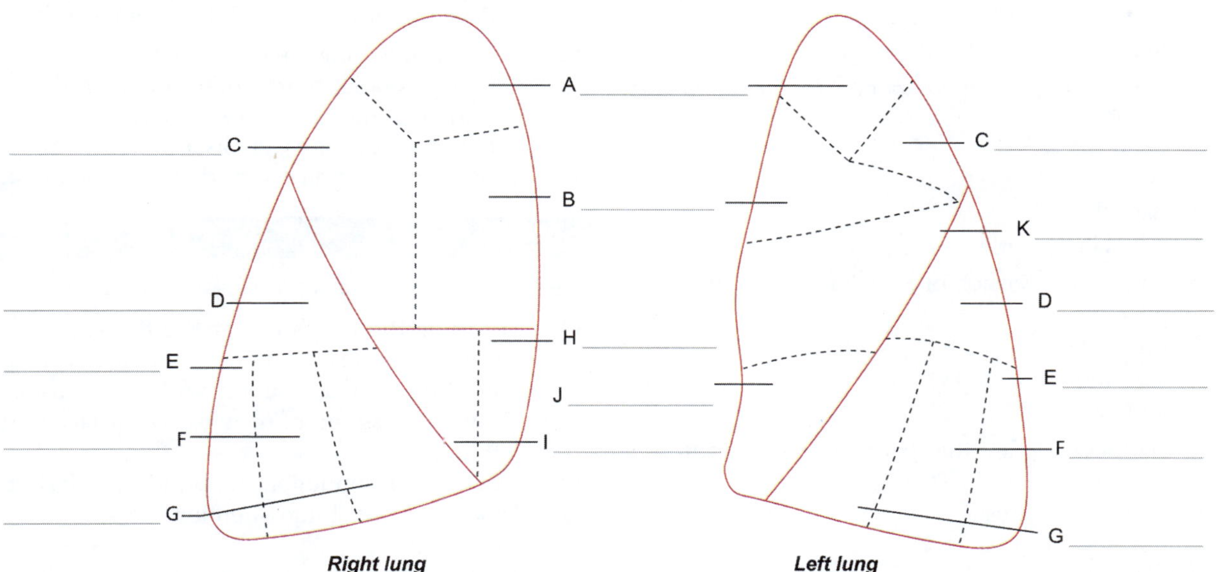

Practice Figure 16.6: The bronchopulmonary segments

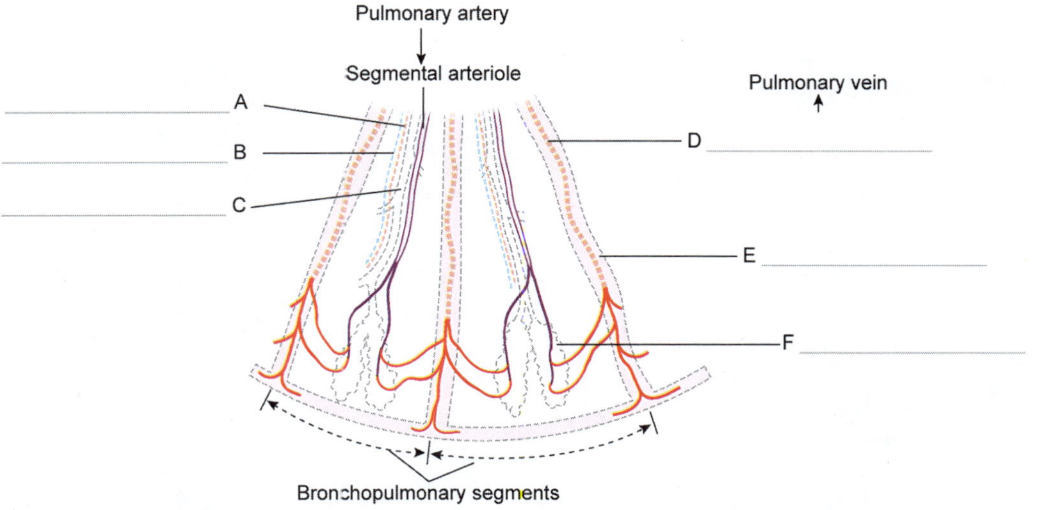

Practice Figure 16.7: Distal portions of adjacent bronchopulmonary segments

MULTIPLE CHOICE QUESTIONS

(Tick the single best correct option)

1. Mediastinal surface of left lung is related to all of the following structures, EXCEPT:
   a. Right atrium b. Oesophagus
   c. Arch of aorta d. Pulmonary trunk
2. The branches of pulmonary artery lie __________ to the bronchus in bronchopulmonary segment.
   a. Dorsolateral b. Dorsomedial
   c. Ventrolateral d. Ventromedial
3. All of the following are true, EXCEPT:
   a. Oblique fissure permits uniform expansion of lung.
   b. Lingula of the left lung corresponds to the middle lobe of the right lung.
   c. Horizontal fissure is present in both the lungs.
   d. Apex lies 2.5 cm above the medial end of clavicle.
4. Pancoast tumour mostly compresses the __________ nerve root.
   a. T1 b. T2
   c. T3 d. T4
5. The right bronchus makes an angle of __________ with the tracheal bifurcation.
   a. 15 degrees b. 25 degrees
   c. 35 degrees d. 45 degrees
6. All of the following are the components of the pulmonary unit, EXCEPT:
   a. Alveolar ducts
   b. Atria
   c. Air saccules
   d. Terminal bronchiole
7. Permanent overdistension of alveoli is known as:
   a. Empyema
   b. Emphysema
   c. Pneumothorax
   d. Dyspnoea
8. All of the following are the structures passing through the root of the left, EXCEPT:
   a. Eparterial bronchus
   b. Pulmonary artery
   c. Pulmonary vein
   d. Bronchial artery
9. Name the structure marked with X.

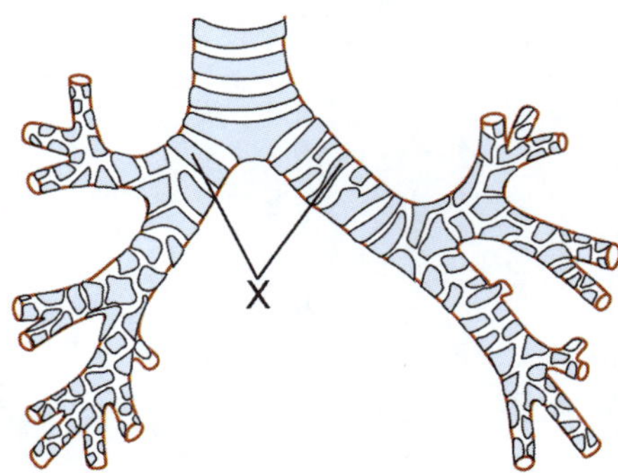

   a. Principal bronchus
   b. Trachea
   c. Lobar bronchus
   d. Segmental bronchus
10. Number of bronchopulmonary segments in superior lobe of each lung is:
   a. 1 b. 2
   c. 3 d. 4
11. __________ segment of lower lobe is the most dependent bronchopulmonary segment in supine position.
   a. Superior b. Anterior basal
   c. Posterior basal d. Lateral basal
12. All of the following are true, EXCEPT:
   a. Foreign bodies mostly descend into right bronchus.
   b. Carina of the trachea is a sensitive area.
   c. Laryngoscopy is a visualisation of interior of trachea.
   d. Bronchial asthma occurs due to bronchospasm.

QUESTION BANK

(Use separate copy to solve the following questions)

Q 1. Describe the lungs under the following headings: External features, relations of the mediastinal surface, blood supply, nerve supply and applied aspects.

Q 2. Draw the diagram of mediastinal surface of right and left lungs.

Q 3. Define bronchopulmonary segment and its importance.

Q 4. What is root of lung? Mention the structures passing through it.

Q 5. Explain: The foreign body enters normally into the right principal bronchus.

eSmartQuiz

Mediastinum

CLINICOANATOMICAL PROBLEM

Clinical Case 1

A 55-year-old male, a chronic smoker for 25 years, presented with progressive swelling of the face, neck and upper chest, along with difficulty in breathing, especially when lying flat. Clinical examination revealed visibly swollen face and dilated veins on the face and neck. Elevated jugular venous pressure was noted. The chest X-ray showed a large mass in the mediastinum, causing compression of adjacent structures, including the trachea and superior vena cava (SVC). The CT scan of the chest confirmed the presence of a centrally located mass in the mediastinum, with associated enlarged mediastinal lymph nodes compressing the SVC. A biopsy confirmed the diagnosis of bronchogenic carcinoma.

1. What is the cause of the SVC compression in this case?
2. What is the anatomical basis for the enlargement of veins of face and neck?
3. In case of SVC obstruction, what is the alternative route of venous blood?

Explanation

1. ______________________________

2. ______________________________

3. ______________________________

PRACTICE FIGURES

(Label the practice figures)

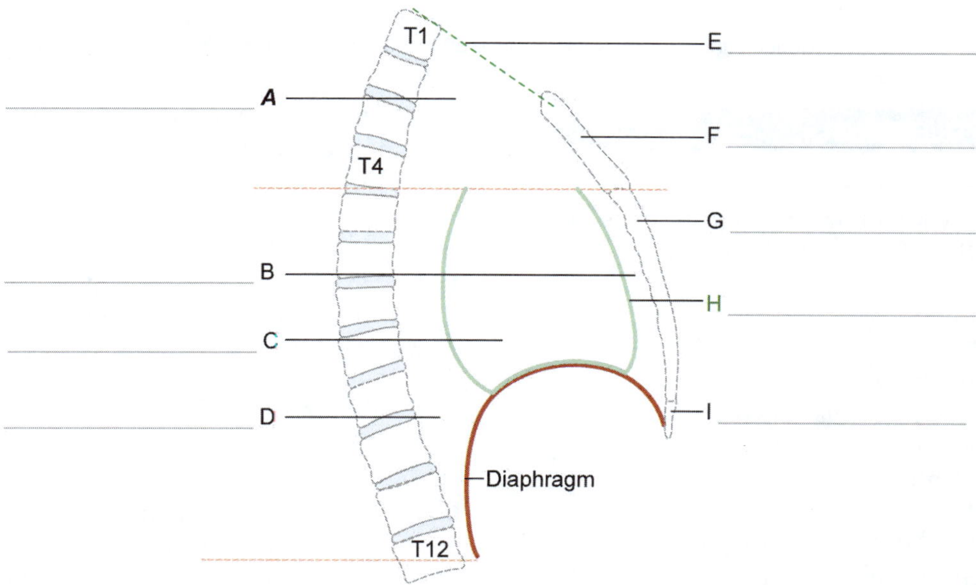

Practice Figure 17.1: Divisions of mediastinum

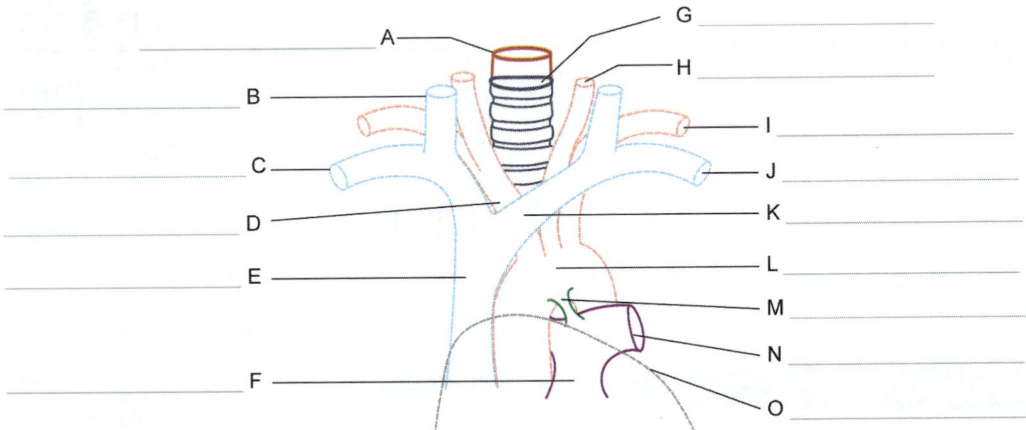

Practice Figure 17.2: Arrangement of the large structures in the superior mediastinum

Note the relationship of superior vena cava, ascending aorta and pulmonary trunk to each other in the middle mediastinum, i.e. within the pericardium. The bronchi are not shown.

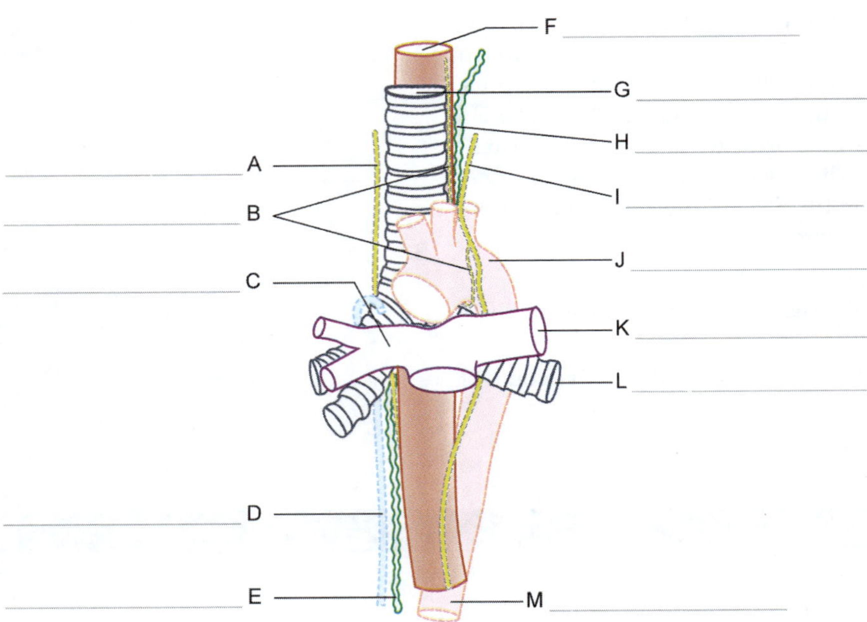

Practice Figure 17.3: Contents of superior and posterior mediastinum

MULTIPLE CHOICE QUESTIONS

(Tick the single best correct option)

1. All of the following are the contents of the superior mediastinum, EXCEPT:
   a. Trachea
   b. Descending aorta
   c. Arch of aorta
   d. Left brachiocephalic vein
2. Boundaries of inferior mediastinum are all, EXCEPT:
   a. Body of sternum
   b. T1 to T4 vertebrae
   c. Diaphragm
   d. Plane passing through sternal angle
3. All structures traverse the whole length of mediastinum, EXCEPT:
   a. Oesophagus
   b. Vagus nerves
   c. Thoracic duct
   d. Trachea
4. All of the following are the contents of middle mediastinum, EXCEPT:
   a. Heart
   b. Ascending aorta
   c. Pulmonary trunk
   d. Trachea
5. The lower part of the thymus gland is located in ______ mediastinum.
   a. Superior
   b. Middle
   c. Posterior
   d. Anterior
6. Which of the following is INCORRECT about the mediastinal syndrome?
   a. Compression of superior vena cava → engorgement of veins of upper half of the body
   b. Compression of trachea → dyspnoea, cough
   c. Compression of oesophagus → dysarthria
   d. Compression of left recurrent laryngeal nerve → hoarseness of voice

7. Which one is NOT a content of posterior mediastinum?
   a. Oesophagus
   b. Descending thoracic aorta
   c. Arch of vena azygos
   d. Vagus nerve

8. ____________ is a content of anterior mediastinum.
   a. Inferior sternopericardial ligament
   b. Arch of aorta
   c. Phrenic nerve
   d. Vagus nerve

9. All of the following are true, EXCEPT:
   a. Prevertebral fascia extends from neck up to the 4th thoracic vertebra.
   b. Pretracheal fascia extends up to and blends with arch of aorta.
   c. Mediastinum is a potential dead space.
   d. In case of lung collapse, mediastinum shifts to opposite the side of the collapsed lung.

10. What is a possible consequence of pus accumulation in the posterior mediastinum?
    a. Referred pain to the shoulders and upper back
    b. Difficulty swallowing
    c. Compression of the thoracic aorta leading to hypotension
    d. Extension of infection into the abdominal cavity

QUESTION BANK

(Use separate copy to solve the following questions)

Q 1. What are the boundaries and contents of superior mediastinum?

Q 2. What are the boundaries and contents of posterior mediastinum?

Q 3. What is mediastinal syndrome?

Chapter

18

eSmartQuiz

Pericardium and Heart

CLINICOANATOMICAL PROBLEM

Clinical Case 1

A 58-year-old male presented to the emergency department complaining of severe chest pain that started about 30 minutes ago. He reported that the pain had been radiating down the medial side of the left arm and forearm and had been associated with sweating and shortness of breath. He denies any recent trauma or heavy lifting. He had a history of hypertension and hyperlipidemia. Clinical examination: The blood pressure 160/90 mmHg, heart rate 100 bpm and respiratory rate 20 breaths per minute.

ECG may showed ST-segment depression and T-wave inversion. The troponin levels were elevated. On evaluation, the clinician considered it as a case of angina pectoris due to myocardial ischaemia.

1. What is the cause of angina pectoris?
2. Why the pain radiated to the left arm and forearm?
3. What is the difference between the angina pectoris and myocardial infarction?

Explanation

1. ______________________________

____

____

2. ______________________________

____

____

3. Angina pectoris: ______________________________

MI: ______________________________

____

____

PRACTICE FIGURES

(Label the practice figures)

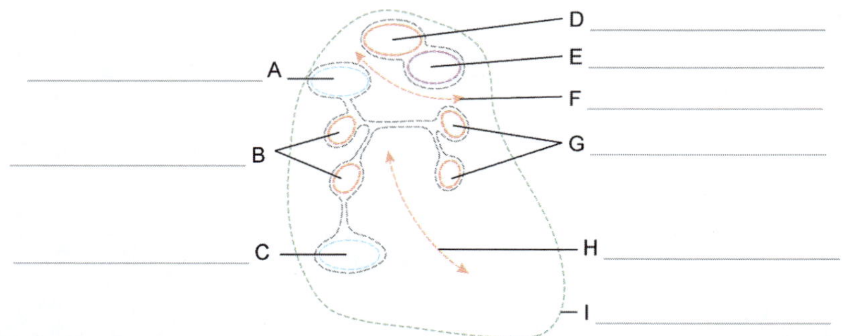

Practice Figure 18.1: Sinuses of pericardium (open pericardial cavity after removal of heart)

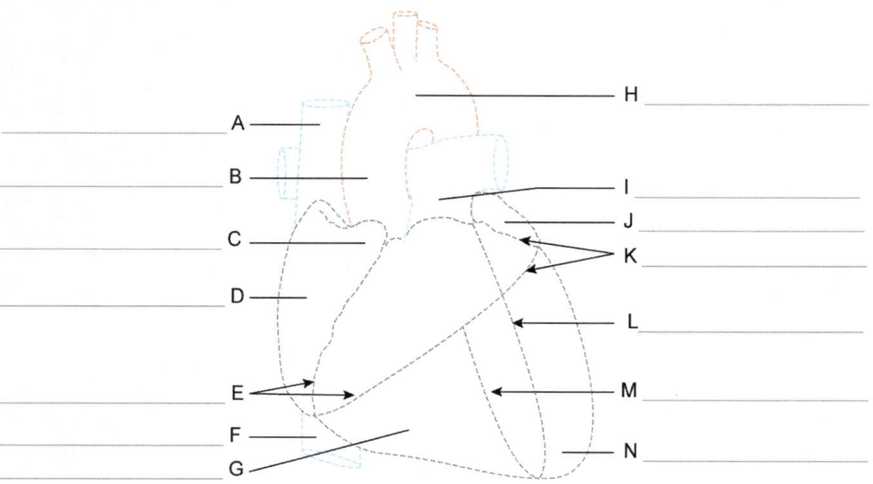

Practice Figure 18.2: External features of heart

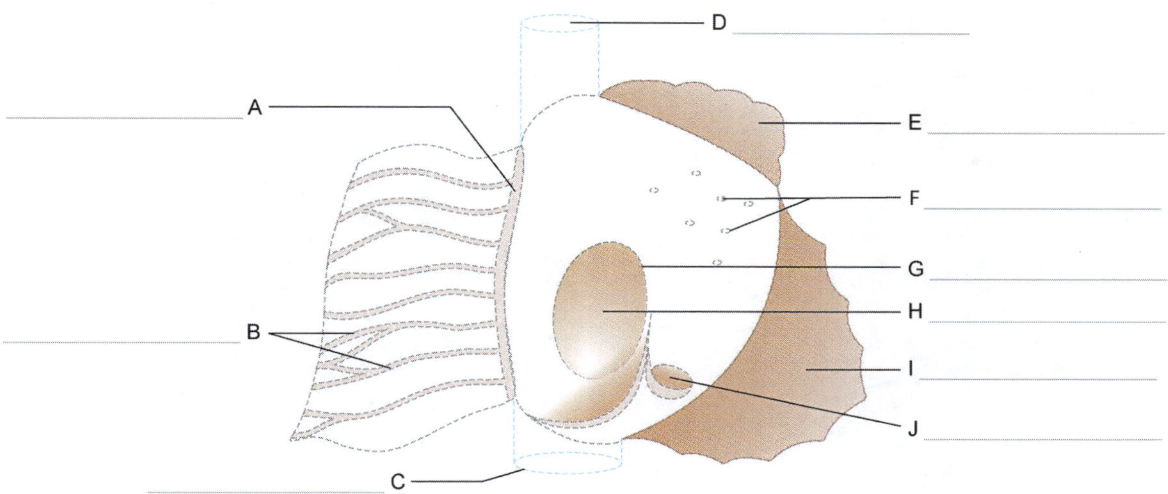

Practice Figure 18.3: Internal structure of right atrium

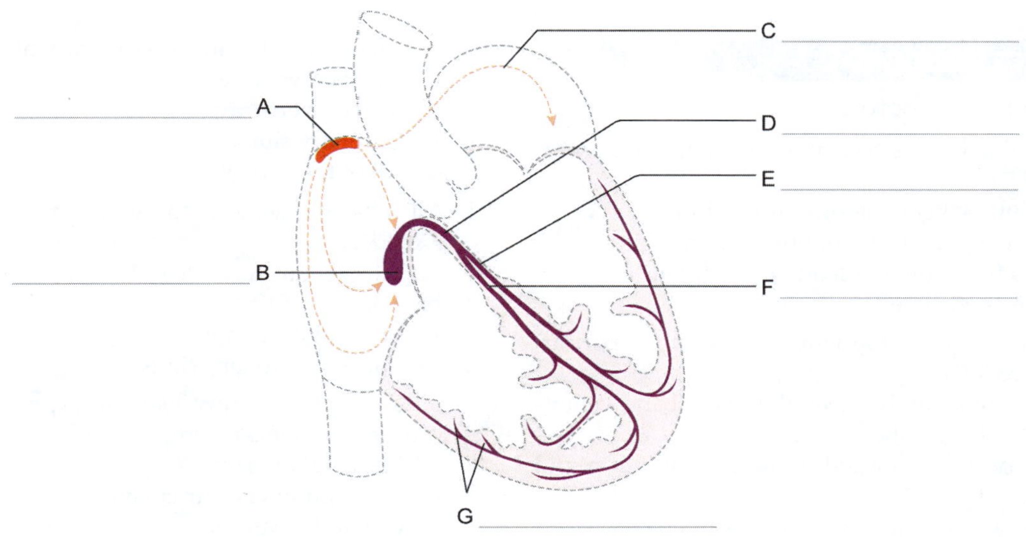

Practice Figure 18.4: Conducting system of heart

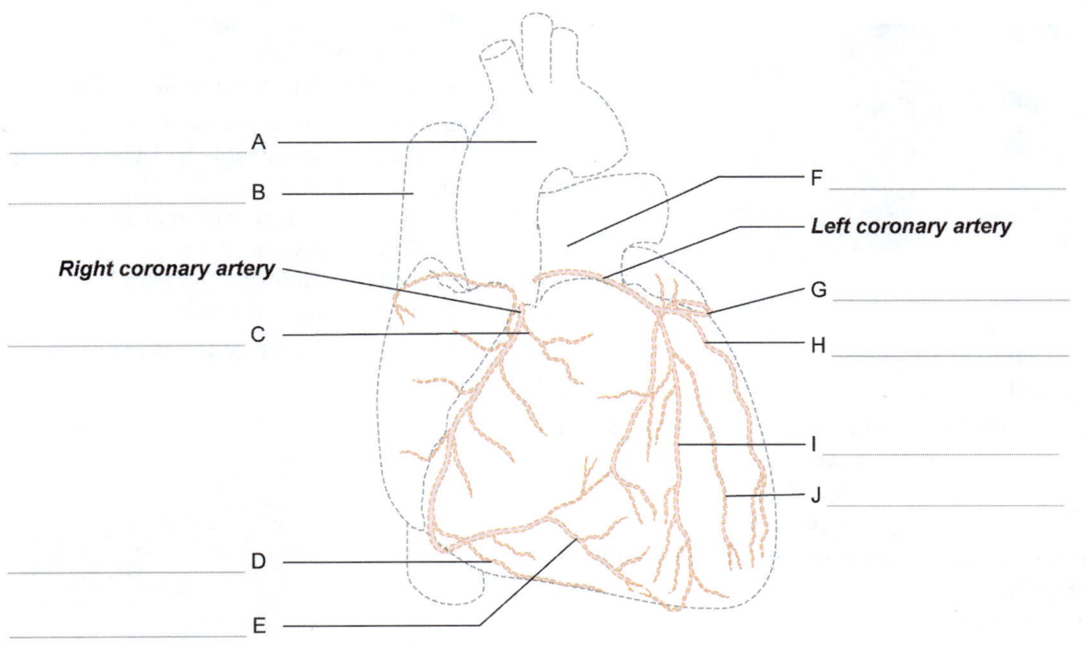

Practice Figure 18.5: Arterial supply of heart

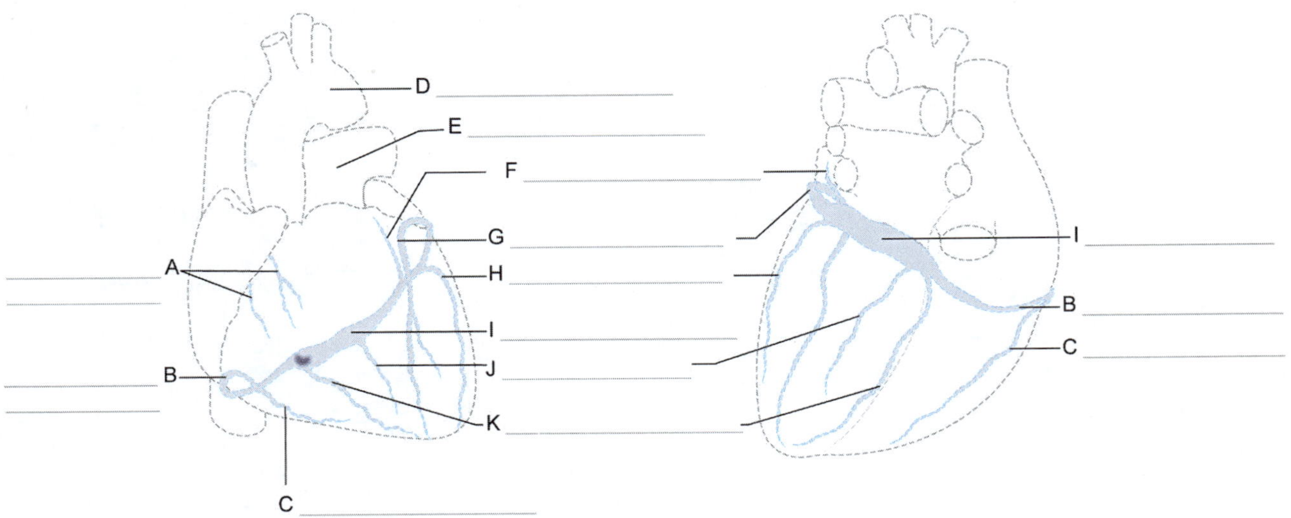

Practice Figure 18.6: Principal veins of the heart

MULTIPLE CHOICE QUESTIONS

(Tick the single best correct option)

1. All of the following are true about the parietal pericardium, EXCEPT:
   a. It is an outer layer of serous pericardium.
   b. It lines the inner surface of fibrous pericardium.
   c. Develops from somatopleuric mesoderm.
   d. It is pain-insensitive.
2. All of the following are true about the transverse pericardial sinus, EXCEPT:
   a. It is horizontal gap between the arterial and venous ends of the heart tube.
   b. Anteriorly it is bounded by ascending aorta and pulmonary trunk.
   c. Posteriorly it is bounded by superior vena cava.
   d. On each side it opens into the plural cavity.
3. Identify the clinical condition shown in the following radiograph.

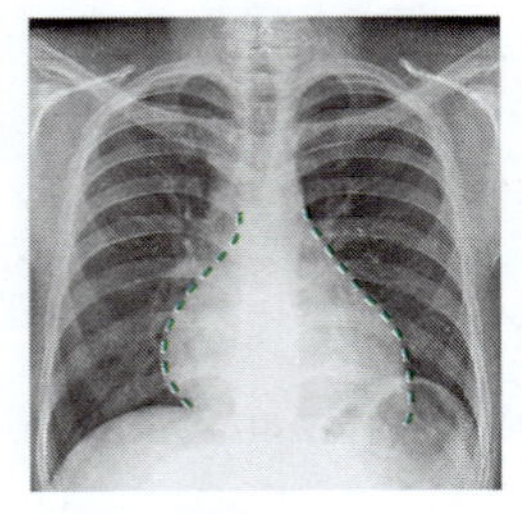
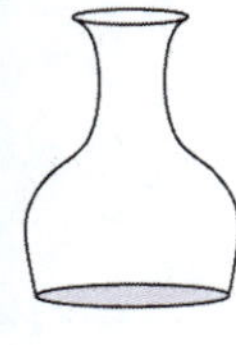

   a. Pericarditis
   b. Pleural effusion
   c. Cardiac tamponade
   d. Pericardial effusion
4. Area of superficial cardiac dullness is seen at left ____________ intercostal spaces.
   a. 3, 4, 5 b. 4, 5, 6
   c. 5, 6, 7 d. 6, 7, 8
5. Sternocostal surface of the heart is mainly formed by:
   a. Right atrium
   b. Right ventricle
   c. Both right atrium and right ventricle
   d. Left atrium
6. Which of the following is a tributary of the right atrium?
   a. Superior vena cava
   b. Inferior vena cava
   c. Coronary sinus
   d. All of the above
7. All of the following are the features of the sinus venarum, EXCEPT:
   a. Intervenous tubercle of Lower
   b. Triangle of Koch
   c. Musculi pectinate
   d. Valve of coronary sinus
8. ____________ is most likely to supply the anterior left ventricular myocardium.
   a. Marginal artery
   b. Posterior interventricular artery
   c. Circumflex artery
   d. Left anterior descending artery
9. The right bundle branch is supplied by:
   a. Right coronary artery
   b. Left coronary artery
   c. Diagonal artery
   d. Anterior interventricular artery
10. Someone suffering a heart attack in his anterior lower right ventricle probably had a blockage in ____________ coronary artery.
    a. Anterior interventricular artery
    b. Circumflex artery
    c. Diagonal artery
    d. Right marginal artery
11. Identify the valve of the heart shown in the following figure.

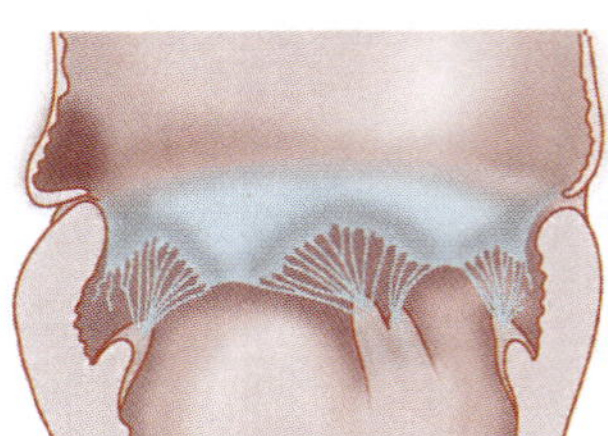

    a. Mitral b. Tricuspid
    c. Aortic d. Pulmonary

12. All of the following are the branches of the right coronary artery, EXCEPT:
    a. SA nodal artery
    b. Right conus artery
    c. Right marginal artery
    d. Anterior interventricular artery

QUESTION BANK

(Use separate copy to solve the following questions)

Q 1. Describe the external and internal features of the right atrium.

Q 2. Describe the origin, course, branches and distribution of right and left coronary arteries.

Q 3. Draw a well-labelled diagrams of:
   a. External features of the heart
   b. Internal features of the right atrium
   c. Internal features of the right ventricle

Q 4. Write a short note on:
   a. Triangle of Koch
   b. Define ischaemic heart disease
   c. Coronary dominance
   d. Sinuses of pericardium
   e. Venous drainage of heart
   f. Cardiac plexus

19 Superior Vena Cava, Aorta and Pulmonary Trunk

eSmartQuiz

CLINICOANATOMICAL PROBLEM

Clinical Case 1

An 8-year-old boy was brought to the pediatric clinic with complaints of exercise intolerance and frequent headaches. He had been feeling tired easily during physical activities such as running and playing sports. His parents reported that his growth had been slower than expected compared to his peers.

On clinical examination, there was a significantly higher blood pressure in the patient's upper limbs compared to the lower limbs (Finding a). Radial and brachial pulses were strong and palpable, but femoral pulses were noticeably delayed and weaker (Finding b). Auscultation of the heart reveals a systolic ejection murmur heard best along the left sternal border (Finding c). The pediatrician diagnosed the case as coarctation of the aorta and advised further investigations.

1. What is coarctation of aorta?
2. Explain the anatomical basis for Findings a, b and c.

Explanation

1. __________

2. Finding a. __________

Finding b. __________

Finding c. __________

PRACTICE FIGURES

(Label the practice figures)

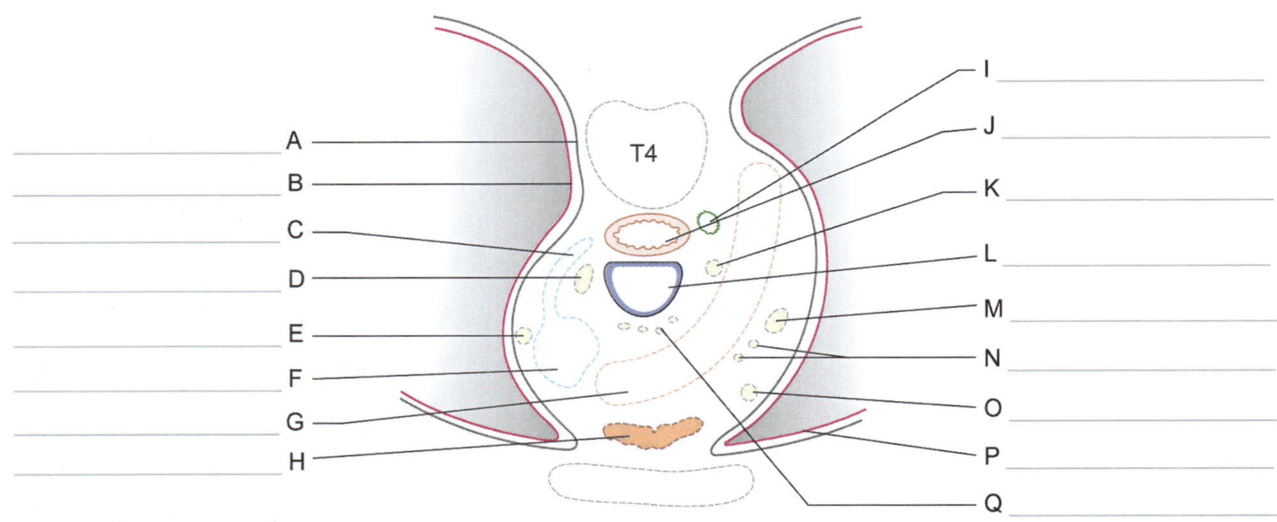

Practice Figure 19.1: Transverse section of thorax passing through the fourth thoracic vertebra (section as visualized from above; faded area is shown for understanding)

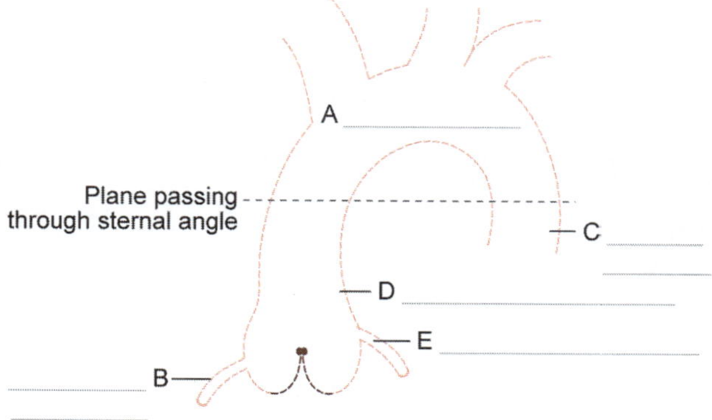

Practice Figure 19.2: Ascending aorta and arch of aorta

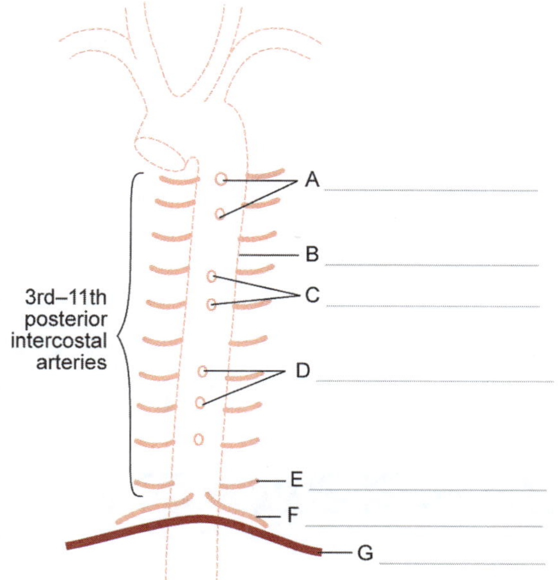

Practice Figure 19.3: Branches of descending thoracic aorta

MULTIPLE CHOICE QUESTIONS

(Tick the single best correct option)

1. All of the following are the tributaries of the superior vena cava, EXCEPT:
   a. Right brachiocephalic vein
   b. Left brachiocephalic vein
   c. Azygos vein
   d. Right subclavian vein
2. All of the following are the tributaries of the brachiocephalic vein, EXCEPT:
   a. Internal jugular vein
   b. Subclavian vein
   c. Vertebral vein
   d. Axillary vein
3. Superior vena cava opens into the right atrium at the level of ____________ right costal cartilage.
   a. First b. Second
   c. Third d. Fourth
4. All of the following are the branches of the descending thoracic aorta, EXCEPT:
   a. Brachiocephalic artery
   b. Subcostal artery
   c. Left bronchial arteries
   d. Superior phrenic arteries
5. Notching of the ribs is observed in ____________.
   a. Coarctation of aorta
   b. Aortic arch aneurysm
   c. Patent ductus arteriosus
   d. Patent foramen ovale
6. Pulmonary trunk bifurcates at ____________ vertebral level.
   a. T2 b. T3
   c. T4 d. T5
7. Aortic knuckle in the radiograph of the PA view of chest is produced by:
   a. Ascending aorta b. Arch of aorta
   c. Descending aorta d. Aortic sinuses
8. Which of the following is the branch of the ascending aorta?
   a. Brachiocephalic trunk
   b. Left common carotid artery
   c. Left subclavian artery
   d. Right coronary arteries
9. Thyroidea ima artery is a branch of:
   a. Arch of aorta
   b. Brachiocephalic trunk
   c. Left common carotid artery
   d. Left subclavian artery
10. Which of the following structures lies anterior to the descending thoracic aorta?
    a. Vertebral column
    b. Hemiazygos veins
    c. Oesophagus
    d. Left lung and pleura

QUESTION BANK

(Use separate copy to solve the following questions)

Q 1. Describe the arch of aorta under the following heading: Beginning, course, relations and branches.

Q 2. Write about the formation, course, tributaries and applied aspects of superior vena cava.

Q 3. Write a short note on:
   a. Ascending aorta
   b. Phrenic nerve
   c. Transverse section of thorax at T4 vertebral level

Chapter

20

Trachea, Oesophagus and Thoracic Duct

eSmartQuiz

CLINICOANATOMICAL PROBLEMS

Clinical Case 1

A 72-year-old male patient came to the OPD with complaints of difficulty in swallowing (dysphagia) and unintentional weight loss over the past few months. He experienced occasional episodes of chest pain and heartburn. He had a history of chronic acid reflux (GERD). Barium swallow showed a rat tail appearance. The clinician diagnosed it as a case of oesophageal carcinoma and advised further investigation after putting a Ryle's tube.

1. What are the normal constrictions of oesophagus felt during insertion of Ryle's tube?
2. What are the causes of dysphagia other than oesophageal carcinoma?
3. Why there is a rat tail appearance on barium swallow in this case?

Explanation

1. a. ____
   b. ____
   c. ____
   d. ____
2. ____
3. ____

PRACTICE FIGURES

(Label the practice figures)

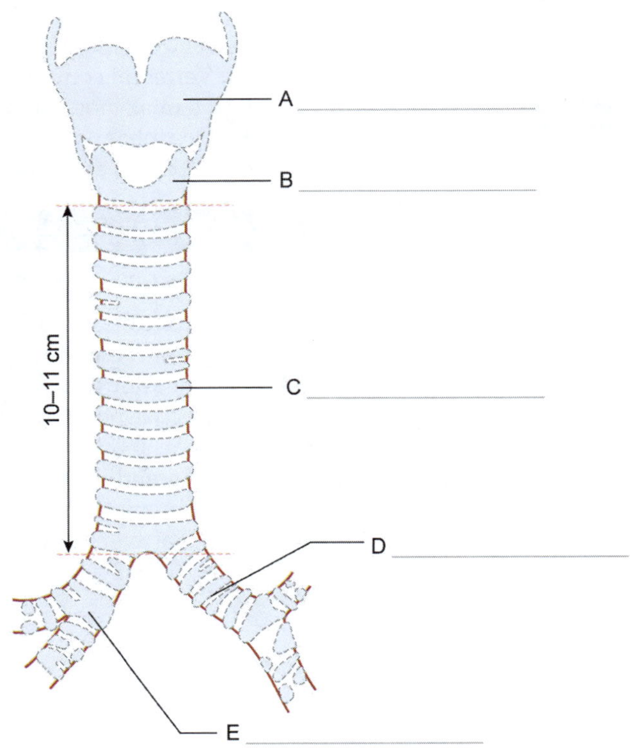

Practice Figure 20.1: Trachea

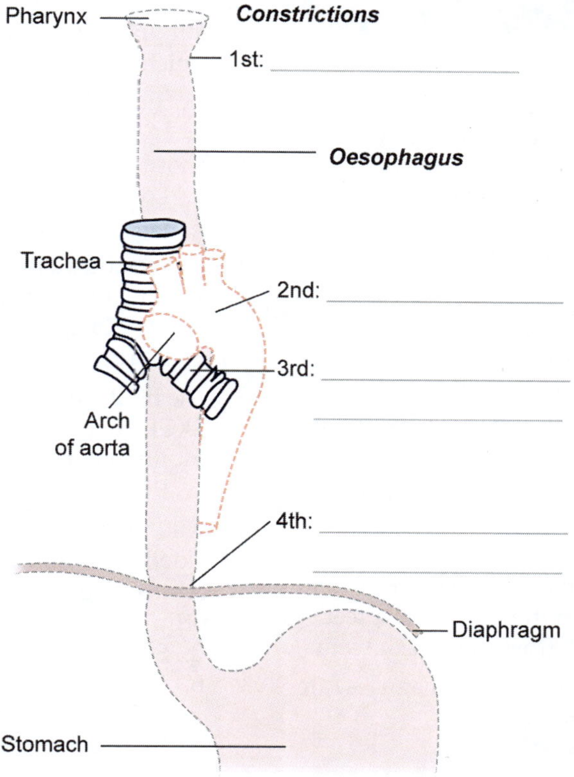

Practice Figure 20.2: Constrictions and parts of oesophagus

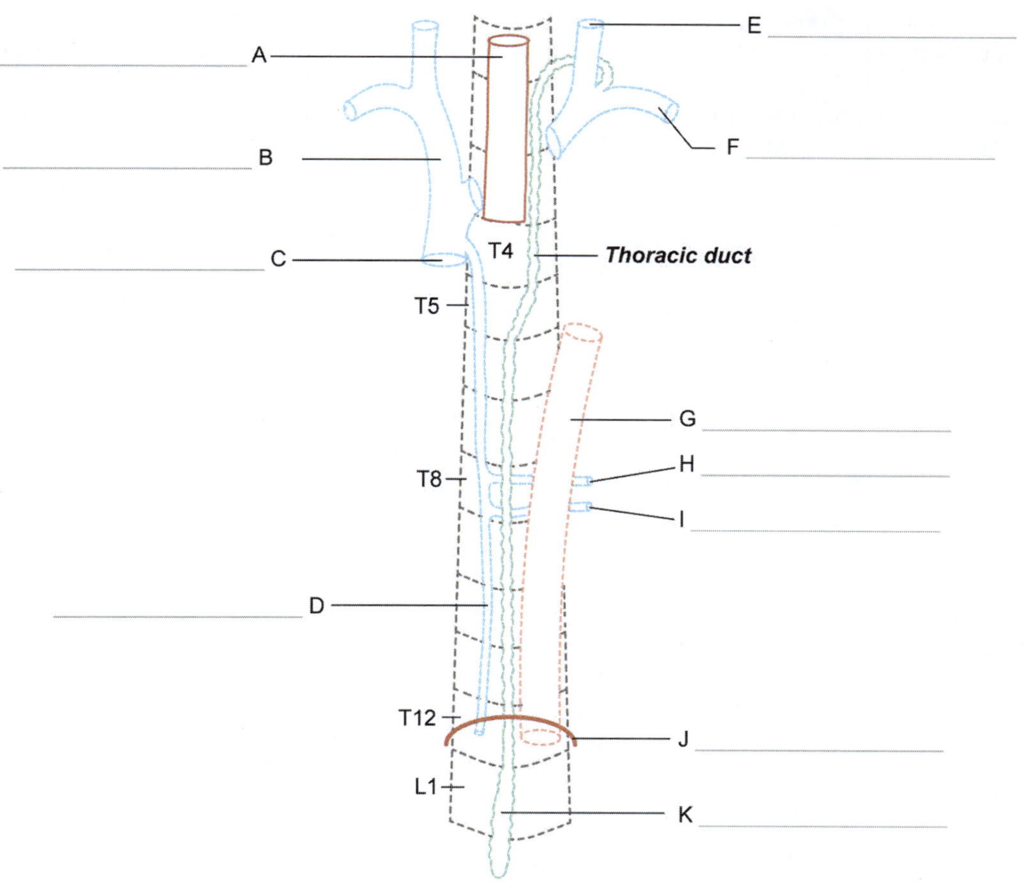

Practice Figure 20.3: Course of thoracic duct

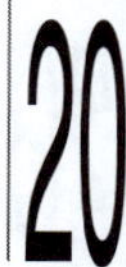

MULTIPLE CHOICE QUESTIONS

(Tick the single best correct option)

1. During childhood, up to the age of 12 years, the lumen of the trachea increases __________ mm per year.
   a. 0.5 b. 1.0
   c. 1.5 d. 2.0
2. All of the following are true, EXCEPT:
   a. In radiographs, the trachea is seen as a vertical translucent shadow.
   b. Tracheostomy is a surgical procedure which allows air to enter directly into trachea.
   c. Carina is present at the beginning of the trachea.
   d. Tracheal mucosa has pseudostratified ciliated columnar epithelium.
3. Which of the following is INCORRECT for the constrictions of the oesophagus?
   a. Fist constriction — 15 cm from the incisor teeth
   b. Second constriction — 22.5 cm from the incisor teeth
   c. Third constriction — 27.5 cm from the incisor teeth
   d. Fourth constriction — 45 cm from the incisor teeth
4. Which of the following part/s of the oesophagus is/are the sites of the portacaval anastomosis?
   a. Cervical
   b. Thoracic
   c. Abdominal
   d. Both a and b
5. Which of the following is INCORRECT for the oesophagus?
   a. Oesophageal mucosa has stratified squamous epithelium.
   b. Portal hypertension may produce oesophageal varices.
   c. Congenital absence of nerve cells in wall of oesophagus results into the achalasia cardia.
   d. In Barrett's oesophagus, the lining epithelium of oesophagus becomes simple squamous epithelium.
6. In mitral stenosis, a barium swallow may indicate the compression of the oesophagus due to enlargement of which structure?
   a. Right atrium b. Left atrium
   c. Left ventricle d. Right ventricle
7. Thoracic duct starts at __________ vertebra.
   a. Lower border of T11 b. Upper border of T11
   c. Lower border of T12 d. Upper border of T12
8. Thoracic duct enter the abdomen through the __________ opening of the diaphragm.
   a. Oesophageal b. Vena caval
   c. Aortic d. Retrosternal
9. The right lymphatic duct drains all of the following areas, EXCEPT:
   a. Right of chest wall b. Right lung
   c. Right of upper limb d. Liver
10. A 40-year-old male complains of a persistent cough with bloody sputum. Upon examination, you suspect a mass obstructing the trachea. Which lymph nodes would be primarily involved in draining lymph from the trachea?
    a. Submandibular lymph nodes
    b. Paratracheal lymph nodes
    c. Supraclavicular lymph nodes
    d. Parotid lymph nodes

QUESTION BANK

(Use separate copy to solve the following questions)

Q 1. Describe the formation, course and termination, relations, tributaries and applied aspects of the thoracic duct.

Q 2. Write a short note on:
   a. Sites of constriction of oesophagus
   b. Trachea
   c. Achalasia cardia
   d. Nerve supply of the oesophagus

Surface Marking and Radiological Anatomy of Thorax

eSmartQuiz

PRACTICE FIGURE

(Label the practice figure)

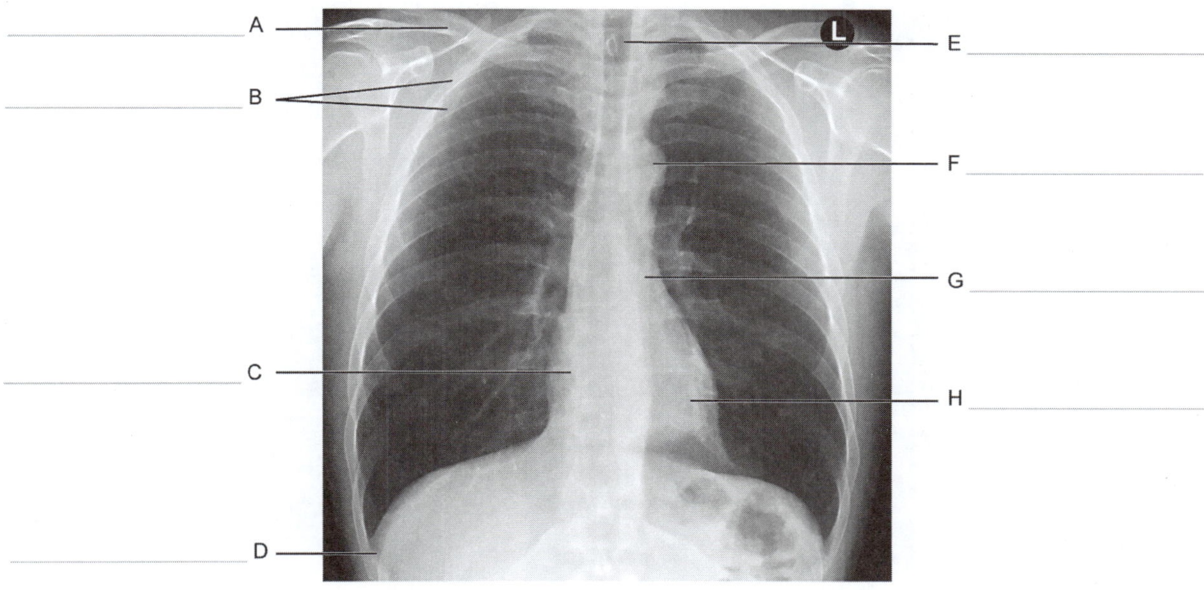

Practice Figure 21.1: Posteroanterior view of the male thorax

MULTIPLE CHOICE QUESTIONS

(Tick the single best correct option)

1. What is the location of the aortic auscultatory area?
   a. 2nd right costal cartilage near the sternum
   b. 3rd right costal cartilage near the sternum
   c. 2nd left costal cartilage near the sternum
   d. 3rd left costal cartilage near the sternum
2. What is the location of the pulmonary auscultatory area?
   a. 2nd right costal cartilage near the sternum
   b. 3rd right costal cartilage near the sternum
   c. 2nd left costal cartilage near the sternum
   d. 3rd left costal cartilage near the sternum
3. The pulmonary trunk extends from upper border of the left 3rd costal cartilage to ____________
   a. Left 1st costal cartilage
   b. Left 2nd costal cartilage
   c. Right 1st costal cartilage
   d. Right 2nd costal cartilage
4. The superior vena cava extends from lower border of the right 1st costal cartilage to upper border of __________.
   a. Left 2nd costal cartilage
   b. Left 3rd costal cartilage
   c. Right 2nd costal cartilage
   d. Right 3rd costal cartilage
5. Which structures chiefly contribute to the formation of the shadow in the mediastinum?
   a. Lungs
   b. Trachea
   c. Heart
   d. Thoracic vertebrae
6. In the PA view of the chest radiograph, the left border of mediastinal shadow is formed all of the following structures, EXCEPT:
   a. Aortic arch
   b. Left margin of pulmonary trunk
   c. Left auricle
   d. Both ventricles
7. In the PA view of the chest radiograph, the right border of mediastinal shadow is formed all of the following structures, EXCEPT:
   a. Right brachiocephalic vein
   b. Superior vena cava
   c. Right ventricle
   d. Inferior vena cava

8. All of the following are correct about the chest radiograph, EXCEPT:
   a. The transverse diameter of heart is half the transverse diameter of the thoracic cage.
   b. During inspiration, heart descends down and acquires tubular shape.
   c. Dark shadow under the right dome of diaphragm due to the gas in the fundus of the stomach.
   d. Arch of aorta produces aortic knuckle.
9. Barium swallow is performed to study __________
   a. Larynx b. Trachea
   c. Oesophagus d. Stomach
10. The rat tail appearance on the barium swallow is seen in case of the __________
    a. Oesophageal carcinoma
    b. Achalasia cardia
    c. Nutcracker oesophagus
    d. Oesophageal compression

Spotters in Upper Limb and Thorax

Answer the questions for the given Spotters or Objective Structured Practical Examination (OSPE).

Note: The purpose of the spotters given here is to orient the students for the practical examination pattern. However, numerous other questions may come for spotters as well. For bone, side determination is important. For muscles, nerve supply and actions are important. For arteries and nerves, their branches are important for spotter examination.

Spotter 1

a. Identify the bone and determine the side.
b. Name the part of the bone marked green.
c. Name the structures attached to it.

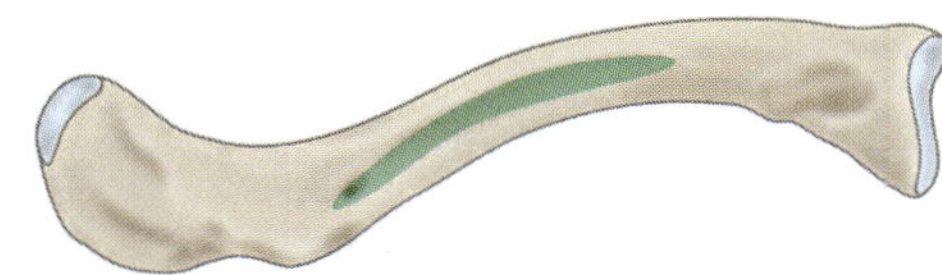

(*Other possible spotter*: Attachments of pectoralis major, deltoid, and trapezius muscles, conoid tubercle, trapezoid ridge)

Spotter 2

a. Name the part of the bone marked green.
b. Name the structures attached to it.
c. What type of epiphysis is it?

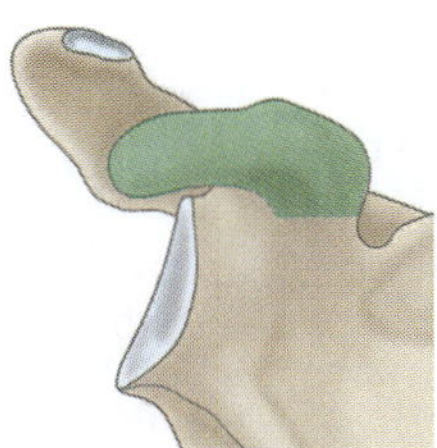

(*Other possible spotter*: Suprascapular notch and structures passing through it, attachments of subscapularis, serratus anterior, long head of biceps brachii and triceps brachii)

Spotter 3

a. Name the part of the bone marked green.
b. Name the structures attached to it.

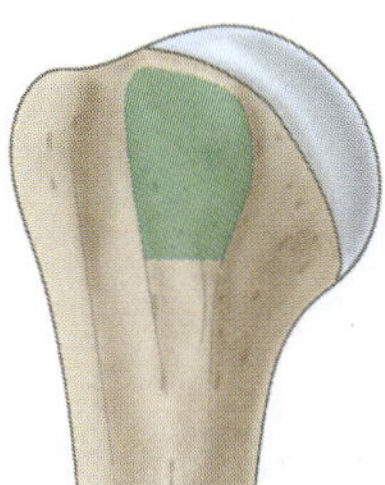

(*Other possible spotter*: Structures passing through bicipital groove and radial groove, deltoid tuberosity and its attachment, nerves related to humerus, attachments of medial epicondyle)

Spotter 4

a. Name the part of the bone marked green.
b. Name the structures attached/related to it.

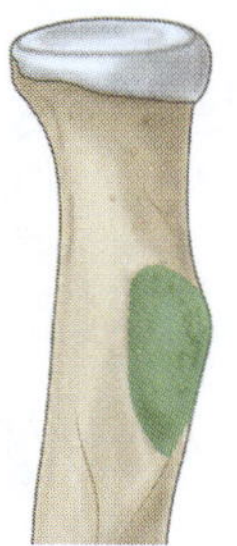

(*Other possible spotter*: For radius: Lister's tubercle and structures related to it, attachment of pronator teres and pronator quadratus. For ulna: Attachments of ulnar tuberosity and olecranon process, groove behind styloid process of ulna)

Spotter 5

a. Name the part of the bone marked green.
b. Name the structures attached/related to it.

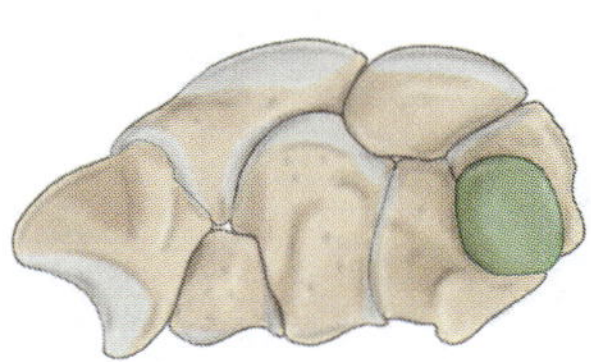

(*Other possible spotter*: Attachment of tuberosity of scaphoid, hook of hamate)

Spotter 6

a. Identify the muscle.
b. Name its nerve supply.

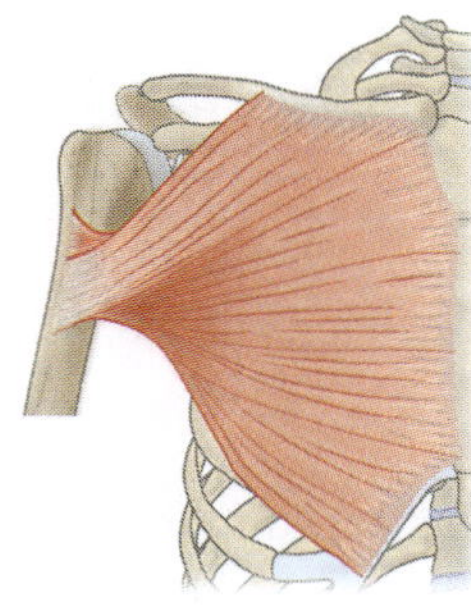

(*Other possible spotter*: Actions of pectoralis major, identification and nerve supply of pectoralis minor)

Spotter 7

a. Name the structure marked with X.
b. Name its branches.

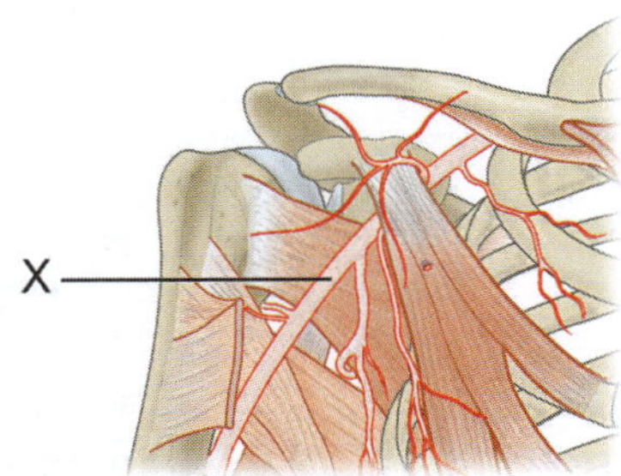

(*Other possible spotter*: Cephalic vein, axillary vein, cords of brachial plexus and its branches)

Spotter 8

a. Name the structure marked with X.
b. Name its branches.

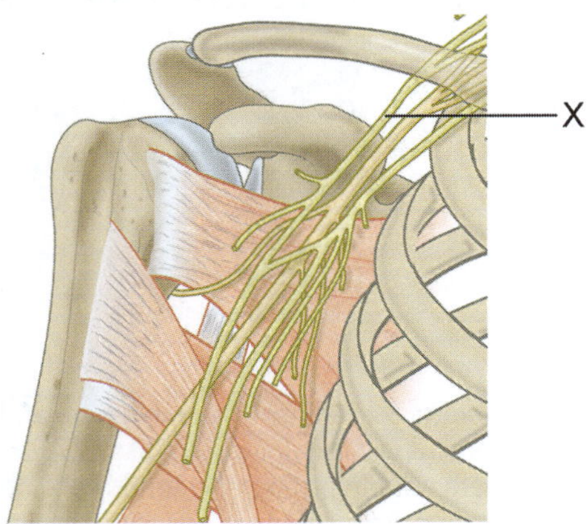

(*Other possible spotter*: Median nerve, ulnar nerve, medial cord, radial nerve, teres major and latissimus dorsi muscles, muscles supplied by specific branch)

Spotter 9

a. Identify the muscle.
c. Name its nerve supply.

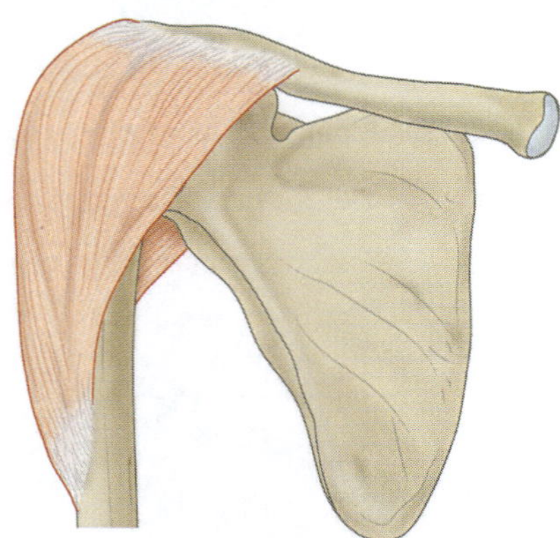

(*Other possible spotter*: Actions, applied, axillary nerve)

Spotter 10

a. Name the structure marked with X.
b. Name its branches.

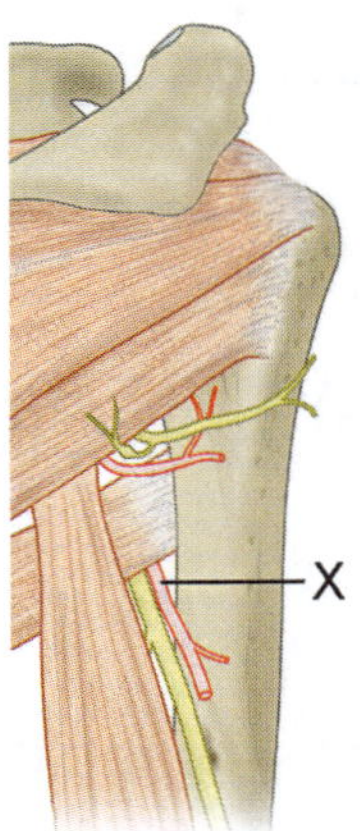

(*Other possible spotter*: Radial nerve and its applied, axillary nerve)

Spotter 11

a. Identify the muscle.
b. Name its nerve supply.

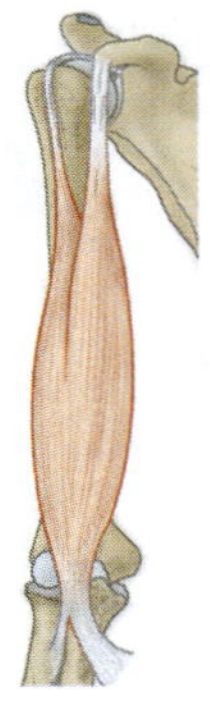

(*Other possible spotter*: Actions and insertion, musculocutaneous nerve and its branches, brachial artery and its branches, triceps brachii–actions, nerve supply)

Spotter 12

a. Name the structure marked with X.
b. Name its branches.

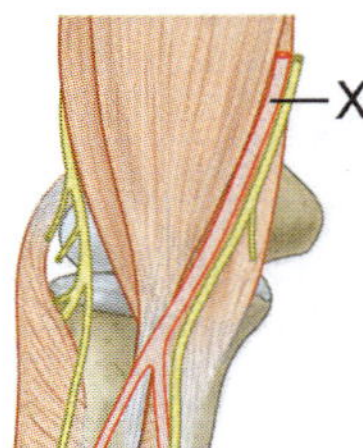

(*Other possible spotter*: Contents of cubital fossa)

Spotter 13

a. Identify the muscle.
b. Name its nerve supply.

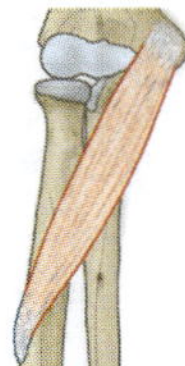

(*Other possible spotter*: Other muscles of anterior and posterior compartment of forearm, radial artery, ulnar artery, ulnar nerve, median and anterior interosseous, radial nerves)

Spotter 14

a. Name the structure marked with X.
b. Name its branches.

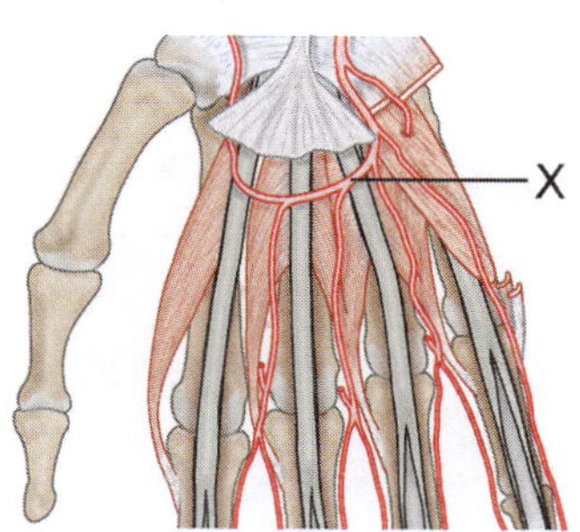

(*Other possible spotter*: Deep palmar arch, deep branch of ulnar nerve, thenar, hypothenar muscles, lumbricals)

Spotter 15

a. Name the structures marked A and B.

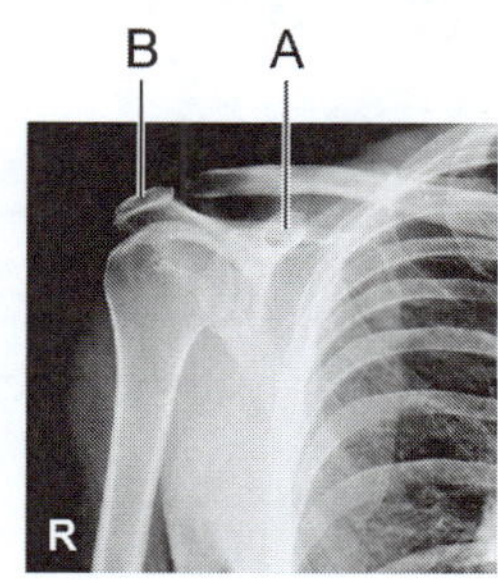

(*Other possible spotter*: Radiographs of elbow region, hand)

Spotter 16

a. Name the part of the bone marked green.
b. Name the structures attached to it.

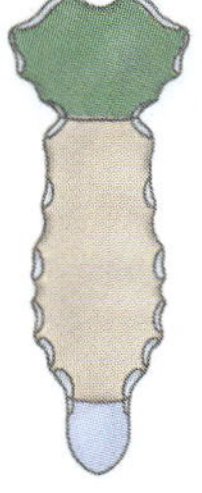

(*Other possible spotter*: Ossification of sternum, xiphoid process)

Spotter 17

a. Name the part of the bone marked green.
b. Name the structures attached to it.

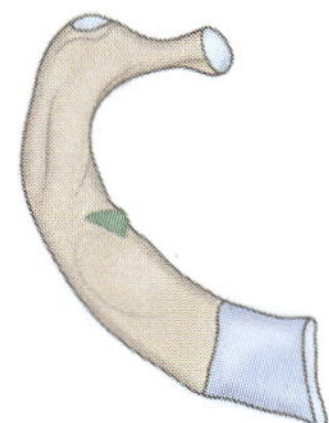

(*Other possible spotter*: First rib: Side determination, relations of the neck, relations of superior surface. Typical rib: Costal groove attachments/relations, 12th rib: Identification, attachments)

Spotter 18

a. Identify the muscle.
b. Name its nerve supply.

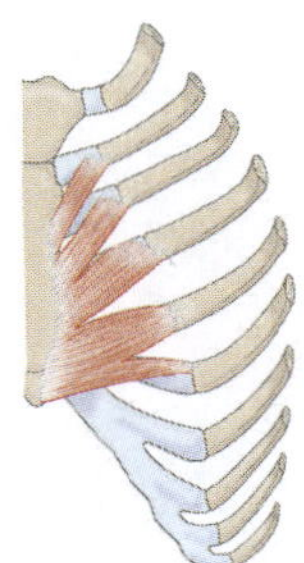

(*Other possible spotter*: Intercostal muscles and their actions)

Spotter 19

a. Name the lobe of the lung marked with X.
b. Name the bronchopulmonary segments of marked lobe.

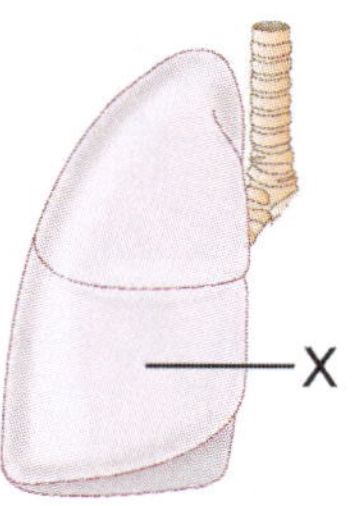

(*Other possible spotter*: Side determination of lungs, mediastinal relations of lungs, structures passing through the root of the lungs)

Spotter 20

a. Identify chamber of the heart marked with X.
b. Name the structures opening into this chamber.

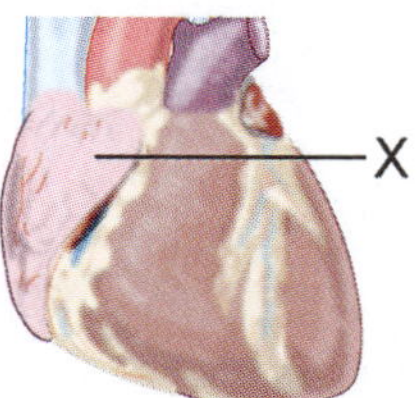

(*Other possible spotter*: Right auricle, left auricle, mitral and tricuspid valve)

Spotter 21

a. Name the structure marked with X.
b. What is its embryological significance?

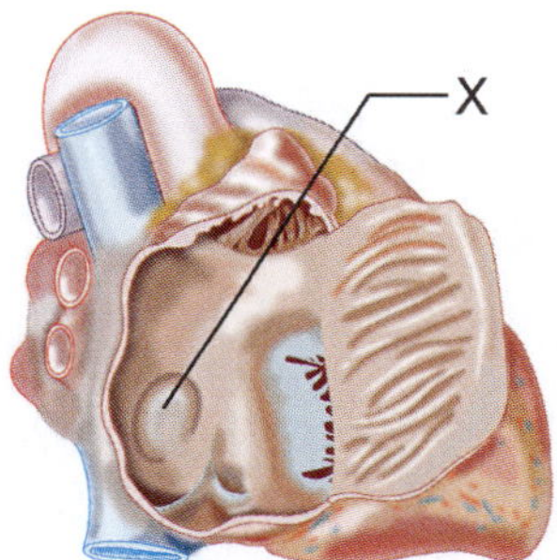

(*Other possible spotter*: Interatrial septum, interventricular septum and their development)

Spotter 22

a. Identify the structure marked with X.
b. List its branches.

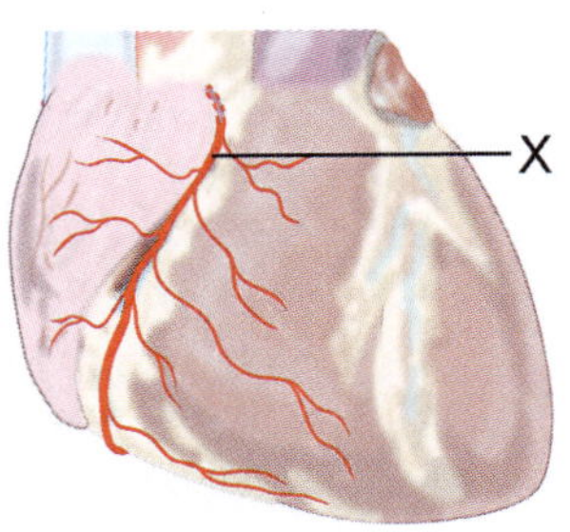

(*Other possible spotter*: Coronary arteries and their branches and area supplied, coronary sinus and its tributaries)

Spotter 23

a. Identify the structure marked with X.
b. List its branches.

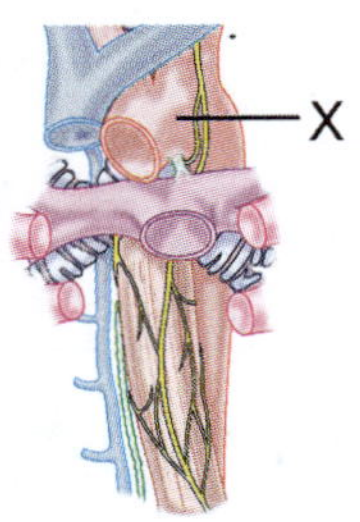

(*Other possible spotter*: Brachiocephalic trunk, brachiocephalic vein, trachea, oesophagus and its constrictions)

Spotter 24

a. Identify the structure marked with X.
b. List its tributaries.

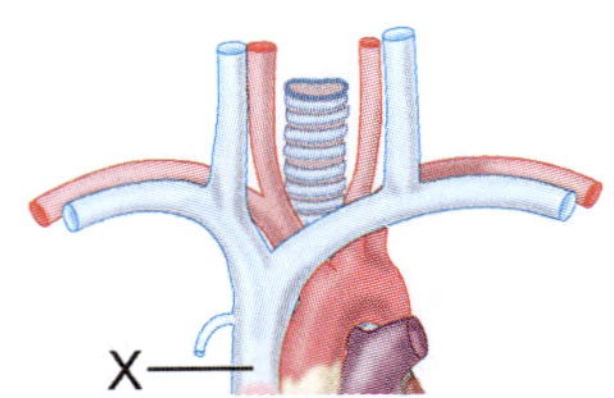

Spotter 25

a. Name the structure marked in the following radiograph.
b. Name the structures above downwards producing left border of mediastinum in the following radiograph.

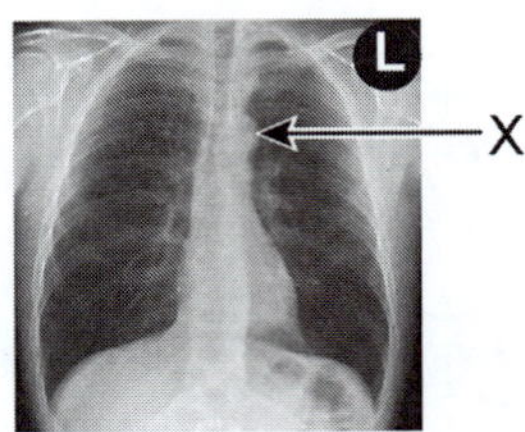

(*Other possible spotter*: Tracheal shadow, pleural effusion, costodiaphragmatic recess, right mediastinal border, cardiothoracic ratio)

Answers

Scan to get key

UPPER LIMB

Chapter 1

Key to Practice Figures

Practice Figure 1.1

A. Clavicle, B. Scapula, C. Humerus, D. Radius, E. Ulna, F. Carpals, G. Metacarpals, H. Phalanges, I. Shoulder, J. Shoulder joint, K. Arm (brachium), L. Elbow joint, M. Forearm (antebrachium), N. Wrist joint, O. Hand (manus)

Practice Figure 1.2

A. Surgical knife (scalpel), B. Cutting edge, C. Surgical blade (size 24), D. Knife handle or scalpel handle (size 4), E. Uses: It is used to cut the skin. It is used to cut the connective tissue, fascia, muscles, vessels, nerves and other structures as and when required.

Practice Figure 1.3

A. Plane forceps, B. Uses: To hold delicate structures such as vessels, nerves and muscles, C. Tooth forceps, D. Uses: To hold the skin and hard structures, E. Pointed forceps, F. Uses: To show the dissected structures during discussion and for fine dissection or to hold thin nerves.

Key to MCQs

1. c	2. c	3. c	4. d	5. b	6. a	7. d
8. c	9. b	10. a	11. c			

Chapter 2

Key to Clinicoanatomical Problems

Clinical Case 1

1. The clavicle gets commonly fractured at the junction of medial two-thirds and lateral one-third. This is the weak point, as it lies at the junction of two opposing curvatures.
2. The shoulder drooped down, because of the weight of the unsupported shoulder.

Clinical Case 2

1. It is a case of winging of scapula of right side.
2. In this condition, the medial border of the scapula became prominent on pushing and punching. The serratus anterior muscle is inserted along the medial border and inferior angle of the costal surface of scapula. This muscle normally helps in stabilizing the scapula against the thoracic wall and assists in protracting the scapula. The winging of scapula occurs due to the paralysis of the serratus anterior muscle.

Clinical Case 3

1. It is a case of a dislocated shoulder.
2. In this condition, the humerus is displaced from its normal position. This displacement results in a dislocated shoulder, where the humeral head has moved out of the glenoid socket, commonly to the anteroinferior aspect of the glenoid cavity.

Clinical Case 4

1. This is the dinner fork deformity that is seen in the Colle's fracture.
2. Due to the trauma, as explained in the given case scenario, there may be a fracture of the lower end of radius with dorsal displacement of the distal fragment leading to a characteristic upward tilt of the hand. It produces a deformity that resembles the shape of a dinner fork when viewed from the side.
3. A plane radiograph of wrist, in anteroposterior (AP) and lateral views, will be helpful for the confirmation of the diagnosis.

Key to Practice Figures

Practice Figure 2.1

A. Sternocleidomastoid, B. Pectoralis major, C. Costoclavicular ligament, D. Sternohyoid, E. Deltoid, F. Trapezius, G. Subclavius, H. Trapezoid part, I. Conoid part, J. Coracoclavicular ligament.

Practice Figure 2.2

A. Pectoralis minor, B. Coracoclavicular ligament, C. Suprascapular ligament, D. Inferior belly of omohyoid, E. Subscapularis, F. Serratus anterior, G. Coracoacromial ligament, H. Short head of biceps brachii and coracobrachialis, I. Long head of biceps brachii, J. Long head of triceps brachii, K. Trapezius, L. Deltoid, M. Long head of triceps brachii, N. Teres minor, O. Teres major, P. Latissimus dorsi, Q. Inferior belly of omohyoid, R. Levator scapulae, S. Supraspinatus, T. Rhomboid minor, U. Infraspinatus, V. Rhomboid major.

Practice Figure 2.3

A. Supraspinatus, B. Subscapularis, C. Pectoralis major, D. Latissimus dorsi, E. Teres major, F. Deltoid, G. Coracobrachialis, H. Brachialis, I. Brachioradialis, J. Extensor carpi radialis longus, K. Common extensor origin, L. Pronator teres, M. Common flexor origin, N. Infraspinatus, O. Teres minor, P. Capsule of shoulder joint, Q. Lateral head of triceps, R. Medial head of triceps, S. Anconeus

Practice Figure 2.4

A. Supinator, B. Biceps brachii, C. Flexor digitorum superficialis, D. Pronator teres, E. Flexor pollicis longus, F. Pronator quadratus, G. Brachioradialis, H. Flexor digitorum superficialis, I. Pronator teres, J. Brachialis, K. Flexor digitorum profundus, L. Triceps brachii, M. Flexor digitorum profundus, N. Aponeurosis for flexor carpi ulnaris, flexor digitorum profundus and extensor carpi ulnaris, O. Extensor pollicis longus, P. Extensor indicis, Q. Anconeus, R. Biceps brachii, S. Abductor pollicis longus, T. Extensor pollicis brevis.

Practice Figure 2.5

A. Scaphoid, B. Lunate, C. Triquetrum, D. Pisiform, E. Trapezium, F. Trapezoid, G. Capitate, H. Hamate, I. Metacarpals, J. Phalanges.

Key to MCQs

1. d	2. a	3. c	4. b	5. d	6. a	7. c
8. a	9. d	10. c	11. b	12. d		

Key to Dissection and Practical Questions

A. Clavicle

For the side determination, hold the clavicle horizontally in such a way that:

1. Its lateral end is flat, and the medial end is large and quadrilateral.
2. Shaft is slightly curved, so that it is convex forwards in its medial two-thirds, and concave forwards in its lateral one-third.
3. Its inferior surface is grooved longitudinally in its middle one-third.

B. Scapula

For the side determination, hold the scapula in such a way that:

1. Its lateral or glenoid (Greek socket) angle is large and bears the glenoid cavity.
2. The dorsal surface is divided by the triangular spine into the supraspinous and infraspinous fossae.
3. Its acute inferior angle is directed downwards.

C. Humerus

For the side determination, hold the humerus vertically in such a way that:

1. Its upper end is rounded to form the head.
2. The lesser tubercle projects from the front of the upper end and is limited laterally.
3. The lower end is expanded from side to side and has a prominent medial epicondyle.

D. Radius

For the side determination, hold the radius vertically in such a way that:

1. Upper end is having disc-shaped head and a narrow neck, while lower end is expanded with a styloid process.
2. Lower end presents a tubercle on the posterior surface called dorsal tubercle of Lister.
3. The medial border of the shaft is the sharpest border.

E. Ulna

For the side determination, hold the ulna vertically in such a way that:

1. Its upper end is hook-like, with its concavity directed forwards.
2. The lateral border of the shaft is sharp and crest-like.
3. Pointed styloid process lies posteromedial to the rounded head of ulna at its lower end.

Chapter 3

Key to Clinicoanatomical Problems

Clinical Case 1

1. The lymph from the upper lateral quadrant drains mainly into the pectoral group of axillary lymph nodes, and later to the supraclavicular nodes. Hence, the clinician should palpate these lymph nodes for the detection of the spread of the carcinoma of the breast.
2. The cancer cells invade the suspensory ligaments, glandular tissue or the ducts. It results in the retraction of the nipple.
3. Mammography helps in the detection of breast cancers.

Clinical Case 2

The anatomical basis for the findings of the clinician are as follows:

1. Breast lump may be due to fibroadenoma or breast cancer.
2. The peau d'orange appearance of the skin is due to blockage of lymphatic vessels, leading to accumulation of lymph and oedema in the skin. It results in the retraction of pits of hair follicles beneath the oedematous skin.
3. The loss of mobility in carcinoma of the breast is due to invasion of deeper structures by cancer cells.
4. Breast cancer commonly spreads through the lymphatic root, mostly to the axillary group of lymph nodes. It causes axillary lymphadenopathy.
5. Breast cancer may spread to the vertebral bodies (breast cancer cells → posterior intercostal veins → vertebral venous plexus → vertebral bodies). These deposited cells form irregular masses in vertebrae.

Clinical Case 3

1. Clavicular head of pectoralis major
2. Sternocostal head of pectoralis major
3. Whole pectoralis major muscle

Clinical Case 4

1. It is a case of winging of scapula of the right side.
2. The serratus anterior muscle normally helps in stabilizing the scapula against the thoracic wall and assists in protracting the scapula on pushing and punching. The winging of the scapula occurred in this case due to injury to the long thoracic nerve, which caused paralysis of the serratus anterior muscle.

Key to Practice Figures

Practice Figure 3.1

A. Axillary tail of Spence, B. Foramen of Langer, C. Breast, D. Nipple, E. Areola, F. Clavicle, G. Subclavius, H. Pectoralis minor, I. Clavipectoral fascia, J. Pectoralis major, K. Pectoral fascia.

Practice Figure 3.2

A. Ligaments of Cooper, B. Lobes (15–20), C. Nipple, D. Lactiferous ducts, E. Pectoral fascia, F. Retromammary space, G. Opening at the tip of nipple, H. Lactiferous sinus, I. Acini, J. Lobule.

Practice Figure 3.3

A. Supraclavicular nodes, B. Apical, C. Central, D. Posterior, E. Anterior, F. Lateral, G. Axillary lymph nodes, H. Posterior intercostal nodes, I. Lymphatics crossing midline, J. Internal mammary nodes, K. Subperitoneal and subdiaphragmatic lymph plexuses, L. Ovary.

Practice Figure 3.4

A. Pectoralis major, B. Clavicle, C. Sternum, D. Costal cartilages, E. Lateral lip of bicipital groove, F. Pectoralis minor, G. Coracoid process, H. From 3rd, 4th and 5th ribs near their costal cartilages.

Practice Figure 3.5

A. Serratus anterior, B. By 8 digitations from upper 8 ribs, C. 1st rib, D. 8th rib, E. 1st digitation on superior angle, F. 2nd and 3rd digitation on the medial border, G. Lower 5 digitations on the inferior angle.

Practice Figure 3.6

A. Clavipectoral fascia, B. Cephalic vein, C. Lateral pectoral nerve, D. Thoracoacromial trunk, E. Lymph vessels, F. Apical lymph nodes, G. Axillary artery, H. Axillary vein, I. Lateral cord.

Key to MCQs

1. a	2. c	3. b	4. d	5. a	6. c	7. a
8. b	9. a	10. c	11. c	12. d		

Chapter 4

Key to Clinicoanatomical Problems

Clinical Case 1

1. There may be damage to the upper trunk of the brachial plexus (C5–C6) at the Erb's point of brachial plexus as a birth injury. This is a meeting point of six nerve: C5 and C6 ventral rami, suprascapular nerve, nerve to subclavius, anterior and posterior divisions of upper trunk.
2. Anatomical basis for:

   Finding a: Impaired function of the deltoid muscle which is innervated by the axillary nerve.

   Finding b: Inability to flex the elbow joint due to weakened biceps brachii muscle, which is innervated by the musculocutaneous nerve.

   Finding c: Inability to supinate the forearm due to paralysis of the biceps brachii (innervated by the musculocutaneous nerve) and supinator muscles (innervated by the deep branch of the radial nerve).

Clinical Case 2

1. The root value of the lower trunk of the brachial plexus is C8 and T1. It is called Klumpke's paralysis/palsy.
2. Anatomical basis for:

   Finding a: The inability to move the right hand and fingers was due to the paralysis of the intrinsic muscles of the hand, including the interossei and lumbricals, which are innervated by the ulnar nerve (C8–T1).

   Finding b: The difficulty in flexing the wrist was caused by the paralysis of the wrist flexors, including the flexor carpi ulnaris and the ulnar half of the flexor digitorum profundus, which are also innervated by the ulnar nerve (C8–T1).

   Finding c: The hyperextended metacarpophalangeal joints and flexed interphalangeal joints represent the characteristic claw hand deformity. The hyperextension of metacarpophalangeal joints occurred due to the unopposed action of the extensor digitorum muscle, while the flexion of interphalangeal joints occurred due to the paralysis of intrinsic muscles of the hand.

Key to Practice Figures

Practice Figure 4.1

A. Posterior: Superior border of scapula, B. Medial: Lateral border of 1st rib, C. Anterior: Posterior surface of clavicle

Practice Figure 4.2

A. Subclavius, B. Pectoral fascia, C. Clavipectoral fascia, D. Pectoralis major, E. Pectoralis minor, F. Axillary fascia, G. Axillary artery, H. Subscapularis, I. Teres major, J. Latissimus dorsi

Practice Figure 4.3

A. Axillary artery, B. 1st part, C. 2nd part, D. 3rd part, E. Humerus, F. 1st rib, G. Subclavian artery, H. Pectoralis minor, I. Teres major, J. Brachial artery

Practice Figure 4.4

A. Axillary artery, B. Thoracoacromial trunk, C. Posterior circumflex humeral artery, D. Anterior circumflex humeral artery, E. Brachial artery, F. 1st rib, G. Subclavian artery, H. Superior thoracic artery, I. Circumflex scapular artery, J. Lateral thoracic artery, K. Subscapular artery, L. Teres major

Practice Figure 4.5

A. Dorsal scapular nerve, B. Suprascapular nerve, C. Nerve to subclavius, D. Lateral pectoral nerve, E. Musculocutaneous nerve, F. Axillary nerve, G. Radial nerve, H. Median nerve, I. Ulnar nerve, J. Medial cutaneous nerve of forearm, K. Medial cutaneous nerve of arm, L. Upper subscapular nerve, M. Nerve to latissimus dorsi, N. Lower subscapular nerve, O. Medial pectoral nerve, P. Long thoracic nerve

Practice Figure 4.6

A. Axillary vein, B. Apical (infraclavicular) nodes, C. Central nodes, D. Anterior (pectoral) nodes, E. Posterior (subscapular) nodes, F. Lateral (humeral) nodes

Practice Figure 4.7

A. Upper trunk, B. Suprascapular nerve, C. Anterior division, D. Posterior division, E. Nerve to subclavius

Key to MCQs

1. d 2. b 3. d 4. c 5. d 6. b 7. c
8. c 9. c 10. d 11. b 12. b

Chapter 5

Key to Clinicoanatomical Problem

Clinical Case 1

1. Trapezius muscle.
2. Paralysis due to injury to the spinal accessory nerve during the lymph node biopsy procedure.

Key to Practice Figures

Practice Figure 5.1

A. External occipital protuberance, B. Ligamentum nuchae, C. Spine of C7, D. Spine of T1–T12, E. Thoracolumbar fascia, F. Medial 1/3rd of superior nuchal line, G. Trapezius muscle, H. Acromion process, I. Scapula, J. Spine of scapula, K. Humerus, L. Latissimus dorsi, M. Iliac crest

Practice Figure 5.2

A. Ligamentum nuchae, B. Transverse process of C1 to C4, C. Spines of C7–T1, D. Spines of T2–T5, E. Medial border of scapula, F. Levator scapulae, G. Rhomboid minor, H. Rhomboid major, I. Scapula

Key to MCQs

1. a 2. d 3. d 4. b 5. b 6. a 7. d
8. c 9. b 10. a

Chapter 6

Key to Clinicoanatomical Problems

Clinical Case 1

1. Axillary nerve.
2. Deltoid muscle which is supplied by the axillary nerve. Its acromial fibres produce abduction at the shoulder joint.
3. The sensory loss over the lower half of deltoid muscle is called regimental-badge area due to injury to upper lateral cutaneous nerve of the arm, a branch of the axillary nerve.

Clinical Case 2

1. Radial nerve.
2. Injury to the radial nerve in the radial groove of the humerus.
3. Weakness of the extension at the elbow occurred due to paralysis of triceps brachii. Radial nerve injury in the radial groove produces partial paralysis of triceps brachii as its long and lateral head receives the innervation before the radial nerve enters the radial groove.

Key to Practice Figures

Practice Figure 6.1

A. Unipennate posterior fibres, B. Intermuscular septum of insertion, C. Lateral 1/3rd of clavicle, D. Crest of spine of scapula, E. Acromion process, F. Intermuscular septum of origin, G. Unipennate anterior fibres, H. Multipennate lateral fibres, I. Deltoid tuberosity of humerus

Practice Figure 6.2

A. Supraspinatus, B. Infraspinatus, C. Teres minor, D. Teres major, E. Humerus, F. Subscapularis

Practice Figure 6.3

A. Axillary vein, B. Axillary artery, C. Axillary nerve, D. Anterior division, E. Posterior division, F Teres minor, G. Pseudoganglion, H. Nerve to teres minor, I. Anterior circumflex humeral artery, J. Surgical neck of humerus, K. Posterior circumflex humeral artery, L. Upper lateral cutaneous nerve of arm

Practice Figure 6.4

A. Acromion, B. Subacromial bursa, C. Supraspinatus, D. Infraspinatus, E. Teres minor, F. Coracoacromial ligament, G. Coracoid process, H. Long head of biceps brachii, I. Glenoid cavity, J. Glenoid labrum, K. Subscapularis, L. Synovial membrane, M. Joint capsule

Practice Figure 6.5

A Circumflex scapular artery, B Long head of triceps brachii, C Teres minor, D Axillary nerve, E Posterior circumflex humeral artery, F Teres major, G Humerus, H Radial nerve, I Profunda brachii artery

Practice Figure 6.6

A Thyrocervical trunk, B Subclavian artery, C Axillary artery, D Deep branch of transverse cervical artery, E Subscapular artery, F Suprascapular artery, G Acromial branch of thoracoacromial trunk, H Ascending branch, I Posterior circumflex humeral artery, J Brachial artery, K Circumflex scapular artery

Key to MCQs

1. a 2. b 3. d 4. d 5. c 6. b 7. a
8. d 9. a 10. c

Chapter 7

Key to Clinicoanatomical Problems

Clinical Case 1

1. Median cubital vein.
2. The median cubital vein is separated from brachial artery by bicipital aponeurosis which mostly prevents the needle from entering the underlying brachial artery. This vein is fixed to deeper veins by a perforator vein.
3. The veins can be made prominent by tying a tourniquet on the arm and asking the patient to do flexion and extension of

elbow. Due to this exercise, the venous return gets increased but is prevented from drainage into deeper veins due to compression applied to the arm. This makes the superficial veins prominent.

Clinical Case 2

1. The lateral and apical groups of axillary lymph nodes.
2. Lateral axillary lymph nodes lie along the upper part of the humerus, medial to the axillary vein. The apical axillary nodes lie deep to the clavipectoral fascia, at the apex of the axilla.

Key to Practice Figures

Practice Figure 7.1

A. Dorsal axial line, B. Ventral axial line

Practice Figure 7.2

A. Cephalic vein, B. Dorsal digital veins of thumb, C. Basilic vein, D. Dorsal venous arch, E. Dorsal digital vein from medial side of little finger, F. Three dorsal metacarpal vein

Practice Figure 7.3

A. Cephalic vein, B. Basilic vein, C. Skin, D. Deep fascia, E. Median cubital vein, F. Bicipital aponeurosis, G. Medial cutaneous nerve of forearm, H. Lateral cutaneous nerve of forearm

Key to MCQs

1. d	2. b	3. c	4. d	5. a	6. c	7. b
8. b	9. b	10. d	11. b	12. a		

Chapter 8

Key to Clinicoanatomical Problem

Clinical Case 1

1. Musculocutaneous nerve.
2. Finding a. Difficulty in flexing the right elbow was due to the paralysis of biceps brachii muscle and brachialis muscles which are supplied by musculocutaneous nerve.
   Finding b. Sensory loss along the lateral aspect of the forearm and hand is due to damage to the musculocutaneous nerve which later continues as lateral cutaneous nerve of forearm.

Key to Practice Figures

Practice Figure 8.1

A. Long head, B. Short head, C. Coracoid process, D. Supraglenoid tubercle, E. Biceps brachii, F. Tendon of biceps brachii, G. Bicipital aponeurosis, H. Insertion: Radial tuberosity, I. Coracobrachialis, J. Insertion: Middle (5 cm) of medial border of humerus, K. Humerus, L. Radius, M. Ulna, N. Origin: Lower half of anterior surface of humerus, O. Brachialis, P. Insertion: Anterior surface of coronoid process of ulna

Practice Figure 8.2

A. Long head: Infraglenoid tubercle, B. Lateral head: Oblique ridge on posterior aspect of humerus, C. Medial head: Posterior surface of humerus below radial groove, D. Posterior part of superior surface of olecranon process

Practice Figure 8.3

A. Profunda brachii artery, B. Posterior descending branch (middle collateral artery), C. Anterior descending branch (radial collateral artery), D. Radial recurrent artery, E. Interosseous recurrent artery, F. Radial artery, G. Posterior interosseous artery, H. Brachial artery, I. Superior ulnar collateral artery, J. Inferior ulnar collateral artery, K. Anterior and Posterior ulnar recurrent arteries, L. Ulnar artery, M. Common interosseous artery, N. Anterior interosseous artery

Practice Figure 8.4

A. Radial nerve, B. Deep branch, C. Superficial branch, D. Ulnar artery, E. Radial artery, F. Median nerve, G. Brachial artery, H. Tendon of biceps brachii, I. Pronator teres

Practice Figure 8.5

A. Lateral: Medial border of brachioradialis, B. Brachioradialis, C. Base: Imaginary line joining epicondyles of humerus, D. Medial epicondyle, E. Medial: Lateral border of pronator teres, F. Cubital fossa, G. Pronator teres, H. Ulna, I Radius, J. Brachialis, K. Supinator, L. Ulna, M. Radius

Key to MCQs

1. c	2. a	3. b	4. b	5. d	6. d	7. b
8. c	9. a	10. a	11. c			

Chapter 9

Key to Clinicoanatomical Problems

Clinical Case 1

1. The pain is due to lateral epicondylitis, also called tennis elbow. This is due to repeated microtrauma to the common extensor origin of extensor muscles of the forearm.
2. It can also occur in swimming, gymnastics, basketball, table tennis, i.e. any sport which involves strenuous use of the extensors of the forearm.

Clinical Case 2

1. Median nerve.
2. Prolonged or repetitive wrist flexion and extension, as seen in activities like typing, may have led to inflammation and swelling of the tissues within the carpal tunnel, causing compression of the median nerve.
3. Tapping over the median nerve at the wrist elicited tingling sensations, known as Tinel's sign.

Key to Practice Figures

Practice Figure 9.1

A. Medial supracondylar ridge, B. Medial epicondyle of humerus, C. Pronator teres (PT), D. Flexor carpi radialis (FCR), E. Palmaris longus, F. Flexor carpi ulnaris (FCU), G. Radius, H. Ulna, I. Pisiform, J. Metacarpals, K. Palmar aponeurosis, L. Anterior oblique line of radius, M. Medial epicondyle of humerus, N. Medial margin of coronoid process, O. Flexor digitorum superficialis, P. Middle phalanges of medial 4 fingers

Practice Figure 9.2

A. Flexor digitorum profundus (FDP), B. Flexor pollicis longus (FPL), C. Pronator quadratus

Practice Figure 9.3

A. Brachial artery, B. Radial recurrent artery, C. Tendon of biceps brachii, D. Supinator, E. Pronator teres, F. Brachioradialis, G. Flexor carpi radialis, H. Palmar carpal branch, I. Superficial palmar branch

Practice Figure 9.4

A. Palmar cutaneous branch of ulnar nerve, B. Volar carpal ligament, C. Ulnar nerve, D. Ulnar artery, E. Flexor digitorum superficialis, F. Flexor digitorum profundus, G. Ulnar bursa, H. Tendon of palmaris longus, I. Palmar cutaneous branch of median nerve, J. Palmar branch of radial artery, K. Median nerve, L. Tendon of flexor carpi radialis, M. Tendon of flexor pollicis longus, N. Radial bursa

Practice Figure 9.5

A. Median nerve, B. Radial artery, C. Palmar aponeurosis, D. Tendon of palmaris longus, E. Ulnar nerve, F. Ulnar artery, G. Palmar cutaneous branches of median and ulnar nerve, H. Palmar branch of radial artery

Practice Figure 9.6

A. Radial bursa, B. Ulnar bursa, C. Digital synovial sheaths

Practice Figure 9.7

A. Tendon of palmaris longus, B. Palmaris brevis, C. Palmar aponeurosis, D. Longitudinal fibres, E. Transverse fibres, F. Superficial transverse metacarpal ligaments, G. Fibrous flexor sheaths

Practice Figure 9.8

A. Lateral cutaneous nerve of forearm, B. Superficial branch of radial nerve, D. Median nerve, C. Ulnar nerve

Practice Figure 9.9

A. Flexor retinaculum, B. Flexor pollicis brevis, C. Abductor pollicis brevis, D. Opponens pollicis, E. Tendon of palmaris longus, F. Palmaris brevis, G. Abductor digiti minimi, H. Flexor digiti minimi, I. Opponens digiti minimi

Practice Figure 9.10

A. Tendon of flexor pollicis longus, B. Tendon of flexor digitorum profundus, C. 4th, D. 3rd, E. 2nd, F. 1st, G. Adduction, H. Abduction

Practice Figure 9.11

A. Radial artery, B. Superficial palmar branch of radial artery, C. Princeps pollicis artery, D. Radialis indicis artery, E. Ulnar artery, F. Deep branch of ulnar artery, G. Deep palmar arch, H. Superficial palmar arch, I. Common palmar digital arteries, J. Palmar metacarpal artery, K. Proper palmar digital arteries

Practice Figure 9.12

A. Median nerve, B. Palmar cutaneous branch, C. Flexor pollicis brevis, D. Opponens pollicis, E. Abductor pollicis brevis, F. Digital cutaneous branches, G. 1st lumbrical, H. 2nd lumbrical

Practice Figure 9.13

A. Anconeus, B. Brachioradialis, C. Extensor carpi radialis longus, D. Extensor carpi radialis brevis, E. Extensor digitorum, F. Extensor digiti minimi, G. Extensor carpi ulnaris, H. Abductor pollicis longus, I. Extensor pollicis brevis, J. Extensor pollicis longus, K. Extensor indicis

Practice Figure 9.14

A. Tendons of flexor digitorum superficialis and profundus with lumbrical, B. Hypothenar muscles, C. Medial palmar septum, D. Midpalmar space, E. Palmar aponeurosis, F. Thenar muscles, G. Flexor pollicis longus, H. Lateral palmar septum, I. Thenar space, J. Intermediate palmar septum

Practice Figure 9.15

A. Anterior interosseous artery, B. Posterior interosseous nerve, C. Extensor pollicis longus, D. Extensor carpi radialis brevis, E. Extensor carpi radialis longus, F. Extensor pollicis brevis, G. Abductor pollicis longus, H. Extensor digitorum, I. Extensor indicis, J. Extensor digiti minimi, K. Extensor carpi ulnaris

Key to MCQs

1. c 2. c 3. a 4. a 5. d 6. a 7. a
8. d 9. b 10. b 11. b 12. c 13. a 14. d
15. c

Chapter 10

Key to Clinicoanatomical Problems

Clinical Case 1

1. Colles' fracture.
2. a. Due to the hand impacts the ground, b. Due to the action of the extensor muscles of the forearm.

Clinical Case 2

1. Anterior (subglenoid) dislocation of the shoulder is common.
2. Plain X-rays can differentiate dislocation of shoulder and fracture of humerus.
3. Axillary nerve as it runs around the surgical neck of humerus.

Key to Practice Figures

Practice Figure 10.1

A. Acromion process, B. Head of humerus, C. Intertubercular sulcus, D. Humerus, E. Coracoid process, F. Glenoid cavity, G. Acromion, H. Coracohumeral ligament, I. Transverse humeral ligament, J. Capsule of shoulder joint, K. Glenoidal labrum, L. Humerus, M. Coracoid process, N. Glenohumeral ligaments

Practice Figure 10.2

A. Acromion, B. Subacromial bursa, C. Supraspinatus, D. Infraspinatus, E. Deltoid (posterior fibres), F. Teres minor, G. Axillary nerve, H. Posterior circumflex humeral artery, I. Long head of triceps brachii, J. Coracoacromial ligament, K. Coracoid process, L. Long head of biceps brachii, M. Subscapularis, N. Glenoid cavity, O. Glenoid labrum, P. Short head of biceps brachii and coracobrachialis, Q. Synovial membrane, R. Joint capsule, S. Deltoid (anterior fibres)

Practice Figure 10.3

A. Radial fossa, B. Capitulum, C. Capsule of elbow joint, D. Olecranon fossa, E. Coronoid fossa, F. Medial epicondyle, G. Trochlea, H. Olecranon process, I. Head of radius, J. Annular ligament, K. Trochlear notch

Practice Figure 10.4

A. Ulna, B. Capsule of elbow joint, C. Humerus, D. Anterior band, E. Posterior band, F. Inferior or oblique band, G. Annular ligament, H. Radius

Practice Figure 10.5

A. Common flexor muscles. B. Flexor carpi ulnaris, C. Ulnar nerve, D. Nerve to anconeus, E. Anconeus, F. Brachialis, G. Median Nerve, H. Brachial artery, I. Tendon of biceps brachii, J. Radial nerve, K. Brachioradialis, L. Extensor carpi radialis longus, M. Extensor carpi radialis brevis, N. Common extensor muscles, O. Annular ligament

Practice Figure 10.6

A. Annular ligament, B. Quadrate ligament, C. Oblique cord, D. Ulna, E. Radius, F. Interosseous membrane

Practice Figure 10.7

A. Ulna, B. Radius, C. Pronation, D. Supination

Key to MCQs

1. a 2. d 3. d 4. b 5. b 6. a 7. d
8. b 9. b 10. b 11. c 12. c 13. d 14. d
15. b

Chapter 11

Key to Practice Figures

Practice Figure 11.1

A. Acromion process, B. Head of humerus, C. Lateral border of scapula, D. Humerus, E. Clavicle, F. Coracoid process, G. Glenoid cavity, H. Ribs, I. Medial border of scapula

Practice Figure 11.2

A. Humerus, B. Olecranon process, C. Head of radius, D. Ulna, E. Radius

Practice Figure 11.3

A. Phalanges, B. Metacarpals, C. Carpal bones, D Radius, E. Ulna

Key to MCQs

1. a, 2. a, 3. b, 4. a, 5. a

THORAX

Chapter 12

Key to Clinicoanatomical Problems

Clinical Case 1

1. The cause of hiccups in this case is irritation of the diaphragm due to GERD.
2. Phrenic nerves.
3. Cause of hiccups: Tumours in the mediastinum, infections, or gastrointestinal disorders, renal diseases, metabolic disorders.

Clinical Case 2

1. Bochdalek hernia.
2. Congenital posterolateral diaphragmatic hernias are more common on the left side.
3. Congenital diaphragmatic hernia of Bochdalek (85–90% of cases).

Key to Practice Figures

Practice Figure 12.1

A. Tip of transverse process of C7 vertebra, B. Suprapleural membrane, C. 1st rib, D. Inner border of 1st rib and its costal cartilage, E. Manubrium

Practice Figure 12.2

A. Inferior vena cava, B. Right phrenic nerve, C. Lateral arcuate ligament, D. Medial arcuate ligament, E. Median arcuate ligament, F. Right crus, G. Left crus, H. Superior epigastric vessels, I. Left vagus (anterior), J. Oesophagus, K. Oesophageal branches of left gastric artery, L. Right vagus (posterior), M. Aorta, N. Thoracic duct, O. Azygos vein, P. Subcostal nerve and vessels, Q. Sympathetic trunk, R. Greater splanchnic nerve, S. Lesser splanchnic nerve

Key to MCQs

1. d   2. d   3. c   4. a   5. a   6. c   7. a
8. c   9. b   10. a

Chapter 13

Key to Clinicoanatomical Problem

Clinical Case 1

1. Thoracic outlet syndrome (TOS) due to cervical rib causes compression of the nerves or blood vessels, often exacerbated by repetitive arm movements.
2. Plain radiograph of the region.
3. Finding a: Muscle wasting in the right hand may be due to long-standing compression of the lower trunk of the brachial plexus.
   Finding b: Diminished pulses in the right upper extremity may be caused by compression of the subclavian artery, leading to decreased blood flow and diminished pulses distally.

Key to Practice Figures

Practice Figure 13.1

A. Clavicular notch, B. Suprasternal notch, C. Manubrium, D. Body, E. Xiphoid process.

Practice Figure 13.2

A. Sternocleidomastoid (sternal head), B. Pectoralis major (sternocostal head), C. Rectus abdominis, D. Costal cartilages, E. Bare area related to pericardium, F. Clavicle, G. Sternohyoid, H. Sternothyroid, I. Area related to pleura, J. Sternocostalis, K. Diaphragm.

Practice Figure 13.3

A. Head, B. Neck, C. Tubercle, D. Costal groove, E. Shaft, F. Costal cartilage

Practice Figure 13.4

A. Scalenus medius, B. Serratus anterior, C. Lower trunk of brachial plexus, D. Subclavian artery, E. Subclavian vein, F. Costoclavicular ligament, G. Sympathetic trunk, H. 1st posterior intercostal vein, I. Superior intercostal artery, J. Ventral ramus of T1 nerve, K. Scalenus anterior, L. Subclavius muscle

Practice Figure 13.5

A. Quadratus lumborum, B. Internal intercostal muscle, C. Diaphragm, D. Lateral arcuate ligament, E. Thoracolumbar fascia, F. Lumbocostal ligament, G. Serratus posterior inferior, H. External oblique, I. Costotransverse ligament, J. Levator costae, K. Erector spinae, L. Longissimus, M. Latissimus dorsi

Practice Figure 13.6

A. Vertebral foramen, B. Spinous process, C. Lamina, D. Transverse process, E. Superior costal demifacet, F. Pedicle, G. Body, H. Superior costal demifacet, I. Inferior costal demifacet, J. Superior articular process, K. Pedicle, L. Inferior articular facet

Practice Figure 13.7

T1: Body – resembles body of cervical vertebrae, Superior costal facet – complete, Inferior costal facet – demifacet, Spine – long and horizontal, T9: Only superior costal demifacet, T10: Costal facet – single circular or oval, T11: Costal facet – single, large circular, extends on to the upper part of the pedicle, No costal facet on transverse process, T12: Body – resembles lumbar vertebrae, Costal facet – single, large oval costal facet, No costal facet on the transverse process, Transverse process with 3 tubercles – superior, lateral and inferior

Key to MCQs

1. b   2. b   3. d   4. a   5. c   6. b   7. b
8. b   9. d   10. a   11. c

Chapter 14

Key to Clinicoanatomical Problems

Clinical Case 1

1. Pott's disease.
2. Localized cold abscess.
3. Cold abscesses lack the typical signs of inflammation, such as heat, redness and tenderness, hence the term "cold." They are characterized by a painless collection of pus formed as a result of the body's immune response to the tuberculosis infection.

Clinical Case 2

1. Thoracocentesis is the procedure to collect the pleural fluid/air.
2. Along the upper border of the rib, not near the lower border.
3. In this case, the 8th intercostal nerve may be damaged as thoracocentesis is performed by inserting a needle along the lower border of the rib. This injured nerve resulted in the patient's complaints.

Key to Practice Figures

Practice Figure 14.1

A. Rib, B. External intercostal muscle, C. Internal intercostal muscle, D. Innermost intercostal muscle, E. Posterior intercostal vessels, F. Intercostal nerve, G. Collateral branches

Practice Figure 14.2

A. Dorsal branch, B. Collateral branch, C. Lateral cutaneous branch, D. Aorta, E. Internal thoracic artery, F. Anterior intercostal arteries

Practice Figure 14.3

A. Posterior intercostal membrane, B. Muscular branches, C. Lateral cutaneous branch, D. Anterior intercostal membrane, E. Anterior cutaneous nerve, F. Dorsal ramus, G. Intercostal muscles, H. Sternocostalis, I. Sternum

Practice Figure 14.4

A. Internal jugular veins, B. Right brachiocephalic vein, C. Superior vena cava, D. Right superior intercostal vein, E. Posterior intercostal veins, F. Right subcostal vein, G. Right ascending lumbar vein, H. Inferior vena cava, I. Thoracic duct, J. Left subclavian vein, K. Left brachiocephalic vein, L. Left superior intercostal vein, M. Left subcostal vein, N. Left ascending lumbar vein, O. Lumbar azygos vein, P. Left renal vein

Key to MCQs

1. a   2. b   3. c   4. c   5. c   6. d   7. b
8. d   9. d   10. a   11. a

Chapter 15

Key to Clinicoanatomical Problems

Clinical Case 1

1. Pleural effusion is the accumulation of fluid in the pleural space.
2. Costodiaphragmatic recess is a potential space located at the junction of the diaphragm and the costal pleura.
3. On chest X-rays, the costodiaphragmatic recess appears at a clear, sharp, well-defined angle where the diaphragm meets the chest wall.
4. Thoracocentesis.

Clinical Case 2

1. Tension pneumothorax is a life-threatening condition characterized by the accumulation of air in the pleural space.
2. The gunshot wound likely allowed air to enter the pleural cavity, which continued to accumulate within the pleural space, but during expiration, the wound may act as a one-way valve, preventing air from escaping.
3. This increased intrapleural pressure shifts the mediastinum away from the affected side.
4. Immediate needle decompression, followed by insertion of a chest tube (thoracostomy). This allows trapped air to escape, relieving pressure within the thoracic cavity.

Key to Practice Figures

Practice Figure 15.1

A. Thoracic wall, B. Cervical pleura, C. Mediastinal pleura, D. Costal pleura (costovertebral), E. Diaphragmatic pleura, F. Costodiaphragmatic recess, G. Diaphragm, H. Sternum, I. Costomediastinal recess, J. Parietal pleura

Key to MCQs

1. c	2. a	3. c	4. d	5. d	6. c	7. a
8. c	9. a	10. b				

Chapter 16

Key to Clinicoanatomical Problems

Clinical Case 1

1. Because the right principal bronchus is wider, shorter and more vertical compared to the left main bronchus, making it more likely for objects to enter into the right lung.
2. Decreased air entry on the right side is due to the obstruction caused by the coin lodged in the right main bronchus.
3. Airway obstruction, aspiration pneumonia, atelectasis (collapse of the affected lung), hypoxemia and respiratory failure.

Clinical Case 2

1. Smoking.
2. Bronchomediastinal lymph nodes.
3. The enlarged bronchomediastinal lymph nodes may exert pressure on the left recurrent laryngeal nerve in the thorax, causing alteration of voice.

Key to Practice Figures

Practice Figure 16.1

A. Upper lobe, B. Horizontal fissure, C. Oblique fissure, D. Lower lobe, E. Trachea, F. Upper lobe, G. Oblique fissure, H. Cardiac notch, I. Lower lobe

Practice Figure 16.2

A. Trachea, B. Right brachiocephalic vein, C. Phrenic nerve, D. Superior vena cava, E. Cardiac impression (right atrium), F. Oesophagus, G. Right vagus nerve, H. Azygos vein, I. Root of lung, J. Pulmonary ligament, K. Inferior vena cava

Practice Figure 16.3

A. Left recurrent laryngeal nerve, B. Thoracic duct, C. Arch of aorta, D. Left superior intercostal vein, E. Root of lung, F. Descending aorta, G. Pulmonary ligament, H. Oesophagus, I. Left subclavian artery, J. Left common carotid artery, K. Vagus nerve, L. Ascending aorta, M. Pulmonary trunk, N. Phrenic nerve, O. Cardiac area (left ventricle, left auricle), P. Lingula

Practice Figure 16.4

A. Eparterial bronchus, B. Pulmonary artery, C. Anterior pulmonary plexus, D. Superior pulmonary vein, E. Hyparterial bronchus, F. Inferior pulmonary vein, G. Areolar tissue, H. Pulmonary ligament, I. Bronchial vessels, J. Posterior pulmonary plexus, K. Bronchopulmonary lymph nodes, L. Hyparterial bronchus

Practice Figure 16.5

A. Trachea, B. Principal/primary bronchus, C. Lobar/secondary bronchus, D. Segmental/tertiary bronchus, E. Terminal bronchus, F. Lobar bronchiole, G. Terminal bronchiole, H. Respiratory bronchiole, I. Alveolar duct, J. Atria, K. Alveolar sac, L. Alveoli

Practice Figure 16.6

A. Apical, B. Anterior, C. Posterior, D. Superior, E. Posterior basal, F. Lateral basal, G. Anterior basal, H. Medial, I. Lateral, J. Inferior lingular, K. Superior lingular

Practice Figure 16.7

A. Bronchial artery, B. Bronchial vein, C. Bronchiole, D. Intersegmental venule, E. Intersegmental plane, F. Alveoli

Key to MCQs

1. a	2. a	3. c	4. a	5. b	6. d	7. b
8. a	9. a	10. c	11. a	12. c		

Chapter 17

Key to Clinicoanatomical Problem

Clinical Case 1

1. The SVC compression in this case may be due to the mass of the bronchogenic carcinoma or enlarged mediastinal nodes.
2. The obstruction of SVC results in the increased pressure in the superficial veins of face, neck and head. This results in dilation and engorgement of veins.
3. Superior vena cava blockage → brachiocephalic veins → subclavian veins → axillary veins → lateral thoracic veins → thoracoepigastric veins → superficial epigastric veins → great saphenous veins → femoral veins → common iliac veins → inferior vena cava → right atrium of heart

Key to Practice Figures

Practice Figure 17.1

A. Superior mediastinum, B. Anterior mediastinum, C. Middle mediastinum, D. Posterior mediastinum, E. Plane of thoracic inlet, F. Manubrium, G. Body of sternum, H. Pericardium, I. Xiphoid process

Practice Figure 17.2

A. Oesophagus, B. Right internal jugular vein, C. Right subclavian vein, D. Brachiocephalic artery, E. Superior vena cava, F. Pulmonary trunk, G. Trachea, H. Left common carotid artery, I. Left subclavian artery, J. Left subclavian vein, K. Left brachiocephalic vein, L. Arch of aorta, M. Ligamentum arteriosum, N. Left pulmonary artery, O. Pericardium

Practice Figure 17.3

A. Right vagus nerve, B. Left recurrent laryngeal nerve, C. Right pulmonary artery, D. Azygos vein, E. Thoracic duct, F. Oesophagus, G. Trachea, H. Thoracic duct, I. Left vagus nerve, J. Arch of aorta, K. Left pulmonary artery, L. Left principal bronchus, M. Descending thoracic aorta

Key to MCQs

1. b	2. b	3. d	4. d	5. a	6. c	7. c
8. a	9. d	10. d				

Chapter 18

Key to Clinicoanatomical Problem

Clinical Case 1

1. Caused by reduced blood flow to the heart muscle, that is, myocardial ischaemia. It occurs due to narrowed or blocked coronary arteries in atherosclerosis.
2. The pain is carried by left-side sympathetic nerves to the T1–T5 segments of the spinal cord. Since somatic nerves (T1–T5) also travel to the same segments, the pain is referred to the skin area. T1 supplies the medial side of arm, forearm and intercostal spaces.

3. The angina is characterized by episodes of chest pain or discomfort that typically last for a few minutes. The pain is usually triggered by physical exertion, emotional stress, or other factors that increase the heart's workload. The pain typically subsides with rest or nitroglycerin. Myocardial infarction or heart attack occurs due to prolonged or complete obstruction of blood flow to a part of the heart muscle, leading to irreversible damage (necrosis) of the myocardium.

Key to Practice Figures

Practice Figure 18.1

A. Superior vena cava, B. Right pulmonary veins, C. Inferior vena cava, D. Ascending aorta, E. Pulmonary trunk, F. Transverse sinus (arrow), G. Left pulmonary veins, H. Oblique sinus (arrow), I. Fibrous pericardium

Practice Figure 18.2

A. Superior vena cava, B. Ascending aorta, C. Right auricle, D. Right atrium, E. Atrioventricular groove, F. Inferior vena cava, G. Right ventricle, H. Arch of aorta, I. Pulmonary trunk, J. Left auricle, K. Atrioventricular groove, L. Anterior interventricular groove, M. Posterior interventricular groove, N. Left ventricle

Practice Figure 18.3

A. Crista terminalis, B. Musculi pectinate, C. Inferior vena cava, D. Superior vena cava, E. Right auricle, F. Openings of venae cordis minimi, G. Annulus ovalis, H. Fossa ovalis, I. Septal cusp of tricuspid valve, J. Opening of coronary sinus

Practice Figure 18.4

A. SA node, B. AV node, C. Bachmann's bundle, D. Bundle of His, E. Left bundle branch, F. Right bundle branch, G. Purkinje fibres

Practice Figure 18.5

A. Arch of aorta, B. Superior vena cava, C. Right conal artery, D. Right marginal artery, E. Inferior (posterior) interventricular artery, F. Pulmonary trunk, G. Circumflex artery, H. Left marginal artery, I. Anterior interventricular artery, J. Diagonal artery

Practice Figure 18.6

A. Anterior cardiac veins, B. Small cardiac vein, C. Right marginal vein, D. Arch of aorta, E. Pulmonary trunk, F. Oblique vein of left atrium, G. Great cardiac vein, H. Left marginal vein, I. Coronary sinus, J. Inferior vein of left ventricle, K. Middle cardiac vein

Key to MCQs

1. d 2. d 3. d 4. a 5. c 6. d 7. c
8. d 9. a 10. d 11. a 12. d

Chapter 19

Key to Clinicoanatomical Problem

Clinical Case 1

1. Coarctation of the aorta is a congenital narrowing or constriction of the aorta.
2. Finding a. The coarctation of the aorta creates a narrowing in the vessel, leading to increased resistance to blood flow distal to the constriction. Blood pressure rises in upper extremities but falls in lower extremities due to aortic coarctation.

   Finding b. The delay and weakness in femoral pulses are due to reduced blood flow beyond the coarctation. However, the pulses in the upper extremities remain palpable and strong because blood flow is maintained through the unaffected arteries proximal to the coarctation.

   Finding c. Systolic ejection murmur heard best along the left sternal border is caused by turbulent blood flow across the narrowed segment of the aorta.

Key to Practice Figures

Practice Figure 19.1

A. Pleura, B. Right lung, C. Azygos vein (terminal part), D. Right vagus nerve, E. Right phrenic nerve, F. Superior vena cava, G. Arch of aorta, H. Thymus, I. Thoracic duct, J. Oesophagus, K. Left recurrent laryngeal nerve, L. Trachea, M. Left vagus, N. Cardiac nerves, O. Left phrenic nerve, P. Left lung, Q. Deep cardiac plexus

Practice Figure 19.2

A. Arch of aorta, B. Right coronary artery, C. Descending aorta, D. Ascending aorta, E. Left coronary artery

Practice Figure 19.3

A. Left bronchial arteries, B. Descending thoracic aorta, C. Oesophageal branches, D. Mediastinal branches, E. Subcostal artery, F. Superior phrenic artery, G. Diaphragm

Key to MCQs

1. d 2. d 3. c 4. a 5. a 6. d 7. a
8. d. 9. a 10. c

Chapter 20

Key to Clinicoanatomical Problem

Clinical Case 1

1. Normal constriction of oesophagus are: a. At its beginning, b. at its crossing by the aortic arch, c. at its crossing by the left bronchus, and where it pierces the diaphragm.
2. Gastroesophageal reflux disease, oesophageal strictures, achalasia cardia, oesophagitis.
3. Due to the narrowing of the oesophageal lumen proximal to the tumour mass, resembling the tail of a rat. It is characteristic of oesophageal carcinoma.

Key to Practice Figures

Practice Figure 20.1

A. Thyroid cartilage, B. Cricoid cartilage, C. Trachea, D. Left principal bronchus, E. Right principal bronchus

Practice Figure 20.2

1st: Pharyngoesophageal junction, 2nd: Crossing of arch of aorta, 3rd: Crossing of left principal bronchus, 4th: At passage through diaphragm

Practice Figure 20.3

A. Oesophagus, B. Right brachiocephalic vein, C. Superior vena cava, D. Azygos vein, E. Left internal jugular vein, F. Left subclavian vein, G. Descending thoracic aorta, H. Accessory hemiazygos vein, I. Hemiazygos vein, J. Diaphragm, K. Cisterna chyli

Key to MCQs

1. b 2. c 3. d 4. c 5. d 6. b 7. c
8. c 9. d 10. b

Chapter 21

Key to Practice Figure

Practice Figure 21.1

A. Clavicle, B. Ribs, C. Right atrium, D. Costodiaphragmatic recess, E. Trachea, F. Aortic knuckle, G. Pulmonary conus, H. Left ventricle

Key to MCQs

1. a 2. c 3. b 4. d 5. c 6. d 7. c
8. c 9. c 10. a

Appendix

Key to Spotters

Spotter 1

a. Clavicle, right side, b. Subclavian groove, c. Insertion of subclavius muscle and clavipectoral fascia

Spotter 2

a. Coracoid process, b. Short head of biceps brachii (origin), coracobrachialis (origin), pectoralis minor (insertion); Ligaments: Coracoclavicular, coracoacromial and coracohumeral. c. Atavistic

Spotter 3

a. Lesser tubercle, b. Subscapularis (insertion)

Spotter 4

a. Radial tuberosity, b. Biceps brachii (insertion in posterior part), synovial bursa (in anterior part)

Spotter 5

a. Pisiform, b. Flexor carpi ulnaris (insertion), abductor digiti minimi (origin), pisohamate ligament, flexor and extensor retinaculum

Spotter 6

a. Pectoralis major, b. Medial and lateral pectoral nerves

Spotter 7

a. Axillary artery, b. Superior thoracic artery, thoracoacromial trunk, lateral thoracic artery, subscapular artery, anterior and posterior circumflex humeral arteries

Spotter 8

a. Lateral cord, b. Lateral pectoral nerve, musculocutaneous nerve and lateral root of median nerve

Spotter 9

a. Deltoid muscle, b. Axillary nerve

Spotter 10

a. Profunda brachii artery, b. Deltoid (ascending) branch, nutrient artery to humerus, radial collateral artery, middle collateral artery

Spotter 11

a. Biceps brachii, b. Musculocutaneous nerve

Spotter 12

a. Brachial artery, b. Profunda brachii artery, superior ulnar collateral artery, inferior ulnar collateral artery, nutrient artery to humerus, ulnar artery, radial artery

Spotter 13

a. Pronator teres, b. Median nerve

Spotter 14

a. Superficial palmar arch, b. Three common palmar digital arteries for adjacent sides of medial 3½ digits, one proper digital artery for medial side of little finger

Spotter 15

a. Coracoid process, b. Acromion

Spotter 16

a. Manubrium, b. Pectoralis major and sternal head of sterno-cleidomastoid muscles (on anterior surface), sternohyoid and sternothyroid (on posterior surface)

Spotter 17

a. Scalene tubercle, b. Scalenus anterior (insertion)

Spotter 18

a. Sternocostalis, b. Intercostal nerves

Spotter 19

a. Inferior lobe of the right lung, b. Superior, anterior basal, lateral basal, posterior basal, medial basal

Spotter 20

a. Right atrium, b. Superior vena cava, inferior vena cava, coronary sinus, anterior cardiac veins, venae cordis minimi

Spotter 21

a. Fossa ovalis, b. The floor of fossa ovalis is developed from septum primum

Spotter 22

a. Right coronary artery, b. Right conus artery, right anterior ventricular branches, right marginal artery, atrial branches, sinoatrial nodal artery, right posterior ventricular branches, posterior interventricular branch

Spotter 23

a. Arch of aorta, b. Brachiocephalic, left common carotid, left subclavian and thyroidea ima arteries

Spotter 24

a Superior vena cava, b. Right and left brachiocephalic veins, azygos vein, mediastinal and pericardial veins

Spotter 25

a. Aortic knuckle, b. Arch of aorta, left margin of pulmonary trunk, left auricle and left ventricle